GIMEL REVIEW
NMC CBT TEST.
UPDATED EDITION.

DISCLAIMER

The author and any other party involved in the production of this work have reviewed all information in this book with resources believed to be reliable, accurate and have made every effort to provide information that is up to date, with best practices as at the time of publication. So therefore, we cannot disregard the possibility of human error despite our best effort and continual changes in best practices the author, publisher, and any other party involved in the production of this book can warrant that the information contained herewith is complete or fully accurate.

The author, publisher and all other party involved in the production of this book disclaim all responsibility from any errors contained in this work and from the results from the use of this information.

Readers are therefore, encouraged to check all information in this book with Institutional guidelines, other resources and up to date information. NMC CBT@ PART 1 TEST is organized by the Nursing and Midwifery Council, United Kingdom, UK and hold no affiliation or support of this product.

GIMEL'S INTRODUCTION

GIMEL Comprehensive Self Study Program! This study is designed to give you Core Contents in a simple easy to understand structure. It will help you identified your strengths and deal with areas of weakness. You will then begin to comprehend many of the major areas of Core contents that are essential to Pass NMC PART 1, CBT TEST.

Whether this is your first attempt or that you have attempted this test several times. I want to encourage you to stay focused on your goals. Cast away feelings of inadequacy and doubt which does not support this effort now. Stay focused and you shall achieve success and your dreams.

This updated edition of GIMEL Study guide with additional contents is a review for International nurses preparing for registration as nurses in the UK.

NMC Test of Competence - Part 1 Test Revision

The NMC Test of Competence Part 1 exam is a computer-based test (CBT) questions consisting of 120 Multiple Choice Questions. It is intended for applicants trained outside the EU (European Union) and European Economic Area seeking employment as a nurse in the UK.

This Part 1 test preparatory review contents covers randomly on all four of the domains and questions specific to adult nursing. These topics are: Professional values, Communication and interpersonal skills, Nursing practice and decision making Leadership management and team working as outlined and stated by NMC.

Thereafter, practice with about 70 questions to test your knowledge with correct answers.

Success is guaranteed if you devote short time to go through the reviewed contents and questions.

This is the opportunity you have been waiting for. Go through the contents. You can be sure of passing your NMC CBT test at First sitting.

Table of Contents

A

Abuse
What is Abuse?
Abuse is when a person hurts another person, either physically, sexually or emotionally. It can happen many times; as such it becomes a pattern. It often continues until the person who is being abused gets help. Sometimes, a friend or family member recognizes the abused and intervene to help.

What are the classifications of Abuse?
It includes: Domestic abuse, Violence abuse, Rape and Sexual Assault.

What does Abuse and Neglect of Vulnerable Adults Means?
It means that, most of the time, older adults are vulnerable to abuse and neglect, especially if they have cared needs.

Warning Signs of Abuse
Neglect: Examples are: Denial of visitors, withholding food, drink, medications, failing to provide their needs. **Warning signs**: Weight loss, bedsores, soiled clothing, complaints of pain or discomfort, dirty or unsafe environment, lack of communication.

Physical: Examples are pushing, hitting, shaking, kicking, grabbing, pulling hair, rough handling, and forced feeding, misuse of medications and inappropriate use of restraint. **Warning signs are:** Unexplained injuries, bruising, unwillingness to seek medical care, changes in the adults' behaviors.

Psychological or Emotional abuse: Examples: Threats to harm, abandonment and neglect, deprivation of contacts, humiliation, blaming, treating someone like a child, threats, intimidation and coercion. **Warning signs**: High blood pressure, low self-esteem, lack of confidence, depression or withdrawal, lack of trust in others, the adult covering in the presence of the abuser.

Sexual: Examples: Being forced to watch pornography or to someone who is in the act physically, rape or sexual assault. **Warning signs**: Pain, irritation or bleeding in the intimate area, difficulty in walking or sitting, torn, stained or bloody underclothes; STIs or pregnancy.

Financial: Examples: Withholding money or possessions, theft, fraud, scam, borrow money and never repay It., pressure on stating or alter some information on Wills, Deeds or Inheritance. **Warning signs:** Unexplained inability to pay for bills or shopping made. Etc. withdrawals of large sum of money, inability to account for any expenses, worry about money, losing money or possessions inexplicably.

Discrimination: Examples: Harassment or maltreatment because of a person's race, gender, disability, age, faith, culture or sexual orientation, bully, threats or unequal care.
Warning signs: The person being used as a scapegoat, denial of access to services, to other service users, lack of respect for religious faith.

Institutional: Poor practices, policies or procedures within a residential home, hospital or day care centre. Routines may be insensitive or don't take into account the unique needs of each person. The needs of the staff are prioritized above the service users. Use of restraint or sensory deprivation e.g. hearing aids is not used.
Warning Signs: No flexibility in the bed time or work routine. Adults been left in the toilet or commode for longer period of time, inappropriate care of the possession or living area, lack of clothes and possessions, inappropriate use of medical procedures, spoken to or referred to disrespectfully.

Respond
Respond when warning signs are observed. Respond sensitively to disclosure.
How to report a concern
1. Get the "Cause Form" concerned or request from your project coordinator as soon as possible.
2. Complete the form, sign and date it.

3. Give the completed form to your Project Coordinator within 24 hours.

Details to include
   a. Include your name and the project or department you are working with.
   b. Name of the alleged abuse and their relationship to the abused
   c. The action taken.
   d. The date, time and location of the disclosure or observation.
   e. Know details of the vulnerable e.g. age, address. Observation to support cause for concern.

Abrasion
What is Abrasion?
Abrasion is a damage or scraped area of skin usually over the bony prominences of the ankle, knee, hip, face and elbow (or ripped off skin).

Accountability
What is Accountability?
- Accountability means that individuals are responsible for their actions and most of the time had to justify them.
- Responsibility means being answerable for one's own actions.
- The NMC (2008) states that
- Nurses and Midwives hold a position of responsibility and other people rely on them. They are professionally accountable to the NMC, as well as having a contractual accountability to their employer and are accountable to the law for their actions.
  (NMC (2008), Accountability Advise Sheet. London, NMC.)
- You must provide a high standard of practice and care at all times.
- Use the best available evidence.

a) You must ensure that any advice you give is evidenced based if you are suggesting healthcare products or services.
b) You must ensure that the use of complementary or alternative therapies is safe and in the best interests of those in your care.

Keep your skills and knowledge up to date.
   a. Ensure to update your knowledge and skills with the current evidenced based practice.

Acid Respiratory Failure

Disorder associated with Acid Respiratory Failure is:

Hypoxemic	Hypersonic
Pneumonia	CNS depression
Pulmonary oedema	Neuromuscular disease
Pulmonary embolism	Acute asthma
Heart failure	Chest trauma
	Pneumo-hemothorax
	Tension pneumothorax
	Spinal cord injury

What are the clinical manifestations of Acid Respiratory Failure?
   a. Change in the level of consciousness or restlessness.
   b. Tachycardia.
   c. Tachypnea (hypoxemia).
   d. Orthopnea.
   e. Hypertension.
   f. Bradypnea (hypercapnia).

And the diagnostics are.
   • Arterial blood gas.
   • Chest x-ray.
   • CBC
   • Sputum culture.
   • Blood culture.
   • Electrocardiogram (EKG or ECG).

Advocacy Services

What is Advocacy Services?

It helps vulnerable people to have access to information and services. They are encouraged to be involved in decisions about their lives, explore choices and options, defend and promote their right and responsibilities and speak out about issues that matters to them.

Airway Obstruction

What are the causes of Airway Obstruction?

Airway Obstruction is a partial or complete blockage of the breathing passage of the lungs.

Causes: -

- Presence of foreign matters
- Allergic reaction.
- Infection.
- Anatomical abnormalities.
- Trauma.

Signs of Oropharyngeal Cancer

1. Persistent sore throat.
2. Difficulty in swallowing.
3. Ear ache.
4. Difficulty in making a speech.
5. Change in voice.
6. Lump in the neck.
7. Painless mouth sore.

Anaphylaxis

What is Anaphylaxis?

Anaphylaxis is a severe and potentially life threatening reaction to trigger an allergy. It develops suddenly and may get worse.

List out the symptoms of Anaphylaxis

- Dizziness.
- Dyspnea.
- Wheezy.
- Palpitation.
- Anxiety.
- Angioedema
- Loss of consciousness.

What do you do if Anaphylaxis emergency situation take place?

1. Call 999 for an ambulance.
2. If trigger is found remove it from the skin.
3. The person should lie down flat: - Except a Pregnant woman, an unconscious patient and If breathing with difficulty should administer adrenaline Injection. Repeat injection after 5- minutes if symptoms did not improve.
4. Adrenaline auto- injectors are Epipen, Emerade jet. These can be very helpful in minimizing the effects of these allergies.

How should someone experiencing Anaphylaxis positioned?

- For pregnant women, may need to lie on their left side or (left lateral) position.
- For someone with dyspnea, placed on fowler's position.
- For an unconscious patient should be placed in the recovery position.

Antibiotic Administration

What are the indications for antibiotic administration?

- Wound that are already showing signs of infection, such pus formation, grey and greenish colouration.
- Wounds of more than 6 hours old unattended to and in need of delayed primary closure.
- Contaminated from humans or animals (e.g. bites).
- Possibilities of inaccessible to deep contaminated wounds (e.g. puncture wounds).
- Exposure to damaged deep tissues.
- Antibiotic should commence after collection of blood sample culture.

Assessment

What is Assessment?

Assessment is the systemic and continuous collection, organization, validation and documentation of information in other to get a complete picture of the patient and how they can be helped.

Which is not part of a cardiovascular assessment?

a. Inspection.
b. <u>Palpation.</u>
c. Percussion.
d. Auscultation.

A full abdominal assessment combines the following in this order;

a. Inspection.
b. Auscultation.
c. Percussion.
d. Palpation.

Palpation: - is used to assess   rebound tenderness, organs and masses and the information needed to be included during the assessment should be mass size, surface(e.g. smooth) , tenderness, consistence, movement and if it has pulse or not.

Percussion – is used to detect air, fluid, faeces, organs and masses.
What are the characteristics of sounds heard on percussion and their examples?

Sound	Examples
• Dull.	Heart.
• Resonant.	Liver, spleen.
• Hype resonant.	No normal organ.
• Tympanic.	Gastric air bubble.

Assignment

Define Assignment?

An assignment is to direct an individual or a group to do activities within an authorized scope of practice. Assignment describes the distribution of work that each staff member is to accomplish in a given work or period.

What are the guidelines for planning assignment?
1. Ensure client safety.
2. Be aware of individual's variations in work abilities.
3. Determines which task can be delegated and to whom.
4. Match the task to the delegate on the basis of the nurse practice scope and appropriate positions description.
5. Provide directions that are clear, concise, accurate and complete.
6. Validate the delegate's understanding of the directions.
7. Maintain continuity of care as much as possible when assigning client care.
8. Communicate a feeling of confidence to the delegated and provide feedback promptly after the task is performed.

AVPU

The **AVPU scale which means; Alert, Voice, Pain, Unresponsive** is a system by which an ambulance crew, first aider or health care professionals can measure and record a patient's responsiveness which indicates level of consciousness.

This is similar to the Glasgow Coma Scale, which assesses a patient's response to Motor skills, Eyes, Voice. The AVPU scale should be assessed using these four identifiable traits, looking for the best response of each.

A - The patient is awake.

V - The patient responds to verbal stimulations.

P - The patient responds to painful stimulation.

U - The patient is completely not responding.

What is the meaning of AVPU?

The AVPU scale has four possible outcomes for recording as opposed to the 13 possible outcomes on the Glasgow Coma Scale. The assessor should always work from best (A) to worst (U) in other to avoid unnecessary tests on patients who are clearly conscious. The four possible Interpretations are:

- **Alert**: The patient is fully awake (although not necessarily oriented). This patient will have spontaneously open eyes, will respond to voice (although may be confused) and will have bodily motor function.
- **Voice**: The patient makes some kind of response when you talk to them, which could be in any of the three component measures of eyes, voice or motor - e.g. patient's eyes open on being asked "Are you OK?" The response could be as little as a grunt, moan, or slight move of a limb when prompted by the voice of the rescuer.

- **Pain**: The patient makes a response on any of the three component measures on pain stimulus, or a peripheral stimulus such as squeezing the fingers. A patient with some level of consciousness (a fully conscious patient would not require a pain stimulus) may respond by using their voice, moving their eyes, or moving part of their body.
- **Unresponsive**: In other words, unconsciousness, this outcome is recorded if the patient does not give any eye, voice or motor response to voice or pain.

A fully alert patient might be considered "alert and oriented very well" if he or she could correctly identify the time, their name, their location, and the event. Health professionals or paramedics may begin with an AVPU assessment, to be followed by a GCS assessment if the AVPU score is below "A."

The Glasgow coma scale is more appropriate in this situation; than the AVPU scale which is not suitable for long-term neurological observation of the patient's state.

What are the limitations?

- It should not be used for long-term follow up of neurological status.
- When compared to the **Glasgow Coma Scale (GCS),** the **AVPU** classification of alertness has been suggested to correspond in the following manner:
A. Alert = 15 GCS;
B. Voice Responsive = 12 GCS
C. Pain Responsive = 8 GCS
D. Unconscious = 3 GCS.

B

Bio- Medical Waste

What is Bio-Medical Waste?

Bio-Medical Waste means any waste which is generated during:

- Diagnosis.
- Treatments.
- Immunization of human beings or animals.
- In research activities or
- In production and testing of biological substances.

Bio- medical waste possess hazard because of its toxicity and infectious.

Blood Transfusion

Why is Blood Transfusion necessary?

It is necessary for:

- Severe iron deficiency or anemia.
- Sickle cell disease or thalassemia.
- Chemotherapy or stem cell transplants.
- Bleeding.

How long does it take to transfuse a pint of blood?

2 - 4 hours, sometimes a little bit faster, but must be cautious.

What is the most important thing to do before blood transfusion start?

Obtain a written consent.

Why is it necessary to run blood at a slow rate?

To prevent fluid overload.

Mention the complications of blood transfusion.
- Back pain.
- Heart palpitation.
- Chills.
- Hyperthermia.
- Difficulty in breathing.
- Restlessness
- Nausea

The unit of blood is usually confirmed by how many nurses?
Two (2) nurses.

To determine a patient's baseline what must the nurse do?
Vital signs must be taken in other to determine the patient's baseline.
How long must you stay with the patient after transfusion is started?
Ideally, 15 minutes.

Body Fluid
List the high risk fluid in the body. They includes:
- Cerebrospinal fluid.
- Pleural fluid.
- Pericardial fluid.
- Synovial fluid.
- Amniotic fluid.
- Semen.
- Vaginal secretions.
- Breast milk.

Breakthrough Pain

What is Breakthrough Pain? It involves:
- **Incident pain** – Pain that can be specifically tied to an activity. An example is change of wound dressing or physical therapy.
- **Spontaneous pain** – It is very unpredictable. This kind of pain cannot be specifically related to time or event of activity.
- **End-of-dose failure** – Pains that occurs at the end of routine analgesic dosing cycle. Specifically when medicated, blood level begins to wear off. This may indicate an increase dose tolerance and may need medication dose alternatives.
- Generally, an analgesic with rapid onset of action within minutes of administration and short duration of action of about 30 minutes is required.

C

Catheterization

What are the reasons for Urine Catheterization?
a. To empty the contents of the bladder. E.g. before and after abdominal, pelvic or rectal surgeries, when necessary.
b. To determine residual urine.
c. To allow irrigation of the bladders.
d. To bypass an obstruction.
e. To reduce or remove retention of urine.
f. To enable bladder function tests to be performed.
g. To measure urine output accurately, for example when patient is in shock.
h. Undergoing bone marrow transplantation or receiving high-dose chemotherapy.
i. To avoid complication during the insertion of radioactive material.

Complications of Catheterization are;
- Retention of urine.
- Fistula formation.
- Leakage of urine around catheter.
- Penile pains on erection.
- Pain intolerance.
- Indwelling catheter.
- Inadequate drainage of urine.

Central Venous Pressure

What does Central Venous Pressure means?
Central Venous Pressure (CVP) is a measurable device for blood volume and venous return. It reflects right-sided filling pressures. It is primarily used to monitor fluid volume status.
Normal values ranges from 2 -8 cm or 2- 6 mmHg.

What are the purposes of measuring Central Venous Pressure?
a. To assess cardiac function by evaluating venous return to the heart.
b. To measure right- sided filling pressures.

What are the likely causes of Increased CVP?

a. Right sided heart failure if the muscle is adequately perform the workload.
b. Constrictive pericarditis or cardiac tamponade.
c. Volume Overload.
d. Pulmonary Hypertension.

What are the causes of Decreased CVP?
- Hypovolemia & Shock.

Chronic Obsessive Pulmonary Disorder

What is the meaning of COPD?

Chronic Obstructive Pulmonary Disorder. It is made up of three other disorders, namely: Asthma, Emphysema, and Bronchitis.

Asthma- An obstructive airway disease caused by spasms and inflammation.

Emphysema- Damage to the air sacs in the lungs.

Chronic Bronchitis - Long term inflammation of the airway.

What are the signs & symptoms of COPD?

- Breathlessness.
- Coughing persistently with phlegm.
- Chest infections.
- Persistent wheezing.
- Weight loss.
- Weakness & tiredness.
- Oedema.
- Chest pain.
- Haemoptysis.or coughing of blood with some sputum.
- The chest of a patient with COPD look like a barrel chest.
- **What are causes of COPD?**
- Whatever the cause may be, COPD occurs when the airways become damaged and inflamed.
- Prolonged cigarette smoking.
- Fumes and dust at work e.g. grain and flour dust, silica dust, welding fumes, coal dust, also cyanides.
- Genetics.
- Air pollution.

What treatment measures are done for COPD?

There is no cure but palliative care.
- Stop smoking.
- Use of inhalers.
- Medications to ease breathing.
- Lung transplant.
- Use of bronchodilator e.g. Beta -2- agonist inhaler and Anti-muscarinic inhaler.
- Long- acting bronchodilator inhalers.
- Steroid inhaler helps reduce inflammation.
- Theophylline tablets or capsules.
- Steroid tablets.
- Antibiotics.
- Pulmonary rehabilitation.

Chronic Kidney Disease

What are the symptoms of Chronic Kidney Disease?

In advanced stage, symptoms may include:
- Tiredness.
- Swollen ankles, feet or hands.
- Shortness of breath.
- Malaise.
- Haematuria.

Causes of CKD are:
- Diabetes.
- High cholesterol.
- Kidney infection.
- Glomerulonephritis.
- Enlarged prostrate.
- Kidney stones.
- NSAIDS.
- Polycystic.

It is a genetic disease that causes cysts to develop in the kidneys.

Palliative treatment for CKD
There is no cure for CKD. The palliative treatments are;
- Dialysis.
- Kidney transplant.
- Lifestyle changes with the control of high blood pressure and high cholesterol.

Clinical Audit

What is Clinical Audit?
- It is the evaluation of performance against established standards of care.
- A quality improvement process that seeks to improve patient care against explicit criteria and the implementation of changes.
- Clinical audit is a very important tool and a quality improvement for the care of patients. Is not a find faulty- tool.
- The clinical audit process will help clinicians decides why they are doing a particular audit and what they want to achieve in carrying out the audit. It would also help one to select the right topic for audit. Good clinical practice or evidence based medicines that are designed for clinical auditors.
- Clinical audits help clinicians formulate measures of quality of evidence for good practices as the basic data collection, develop data collection, protocols and tools. Advance on data collection on clinical audits ensures patient confidentiality, as well as data protection issued and addressed.
- The clinical audit will help one to understand the use of statistics for analyzing and presenting of data collection, which helps clinicians to analyze course of problem and how they improve quality of care. It will also help clinicians manage review, together with the findings made with their colleagues and be able to prepare clinical audit reports.

Who are the target audience?
They are:
(1)Surgeons (2) Obstetricians and Gynecologists (3) Anesthetists, (4) Nurses (5) Pharmacists, (6) Microbiologists (7) Administrators (8) Infection Controllers (9) Physicians, (10) Quality Managers.

Definition of Clinical Audit; It is a frame work through which NHS organization are accountable for continually improving the quality of their services, safeguarding high standard of care by creating an enabling environment in which excellent clinical care will flourish.

Audit Cycle.

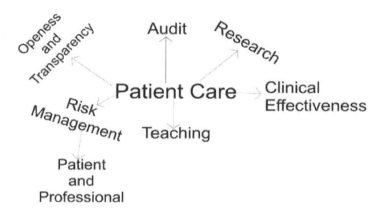

Clinical Benchmarking

Benchmarking is a comparison and measurement of a healthcare organization's services against other national healthcare organizations. It provides leaders with insight to help them understand how their organization works are compared with similar a organization that provides the same services. It also allows for the sharing of best practices and evidenced-based practice (EBP), clinical research outcomes between healthcare facilities at a national level. Benchmarks can be tailored to specific areas of nursing, such as acute and long term care hospitals, hospice, and home health facilities. The four core principles of clinical practice benchmarking are: maintaining quality of services, improving customer satisfaction, improving patient safety, and continuous improvement.

Colostomy

A colostomy is an opening (stoma) found in the large in the large intestine.

What conditions/ Indications required Colostomy for treatments?

- Colorectal cancers.
- Crohn's disease.
- Diverticulitis.
- Vaginal or cervical cancers.
- Bowel incontinence.
- Gangrenous Sigmoid Volvulus
- Hirschsprung's disease.

What are the types of Colostomies?

a. Loop colostomy - A loop of colon is pulled out through a stoma. It is temporary.
b. End colostomy- Is often permanent.
c. Double barrel colostomy. - The bowel has both ends which are brought out to abdomen. It is a temporary colostomy with two openings that occurs through the proximal stoma.

The Stoma: is usually on the left-hand side of the abdomen. The characteristic of a stoma involves reddish, moist and sometimes bloody stoma. It is not painful. Stomas vary in shape, size, and some are flat while some are in a circular form. A stoma is the side of the abdomen where the tube is inserted. No sensation and no pain.

Communication

What is Communication? A model in which health workers and nurses conduct a structured and evidence based conversation. Two categories are SAGE & THYME.

What is the full meaning of SAGE & THYME?

- S- Setting.
- Ask.
- G- Gather.
- E- Empathy.
- T- Talk.
- H- Help.
- Y- You.
- M- Me.
- E- End.

What are the barriers to communication?
- Poor memory.
- Reduced concentration and short attention span.
- Distractibility.
- Generalized fatigue.

The barriers to effective communication are;
- Poor communication with patient can negatively affect decision making.
- Environmental conditions.
- Personal emotional disturbances.
- The Impact when providing a supportive role to patient with psychological and emotional issues.
- Institutions work environment and inability to adapt can influence communication.
- When communicating and assessing patient needs, nurses may be anxious about eliciting distress and managing expressed concerns.
- Lack of Confidentiality and inappropriate disclosure of information about the patient.

- Inability to process language and accent differences.

The elements of non-verbal responses are; SOLER
- S- Face the patient squarely.
- O- Maintain an Open posture.
- L- Leaning slightly towards the patient to convey interest.
- E- Eye contact should be appropriate.
- R- Relaxed.

What is Interpersonal Communication?
It is the process of discussion between health care professional, patient and care givers in other to explore issue and arrive at positive conclusions.

What are the essential features of maintaining dignity in Communication?
- Attitude.
- Behavior.
- Compassion.
- Dialogue.

Communication Disorder

Aphasia- is an acquired communication disorder that impairs a person's ability to process language and not speech impairment caused by damage to the muscles involved with speech.
- **Dysarthria-** is a motor speech disorder, as a result of neurological or muscular changes, causing difficulty in producing speed and co-ordination of the movement needed to achieve appropriate and articulation for speech.
- **Dyspraxia-** speech disorders that is not caused by muscles weakness or sensory loss but a disorder of initiating and sequencing purposeful voluntary movement.
- **Dysphoria-** mood variation, grief reaction and dissatisfied with life. More of a mental disorder.

Compartment Syndrome

What is Compartment Syndrome?

Compartment Syndrome is a painful and serious condition caused by bleeding or swelling within an enclosed bundle of muscles compartment.
 Compartment syndrome occurs when the pressure within a compartment increases, restricting the blood flow to the area and potentially damaging the muscles and nearby nerves. It usually occurs in the legs, feet, arms or hands, but can occur wherever there's an enclosed compartment inside the body.

What are the types of Compartment Syndrome?
There are two main types:
Acute and Chronic Compartment Syndrome.

Acute Compartment Syndrome – happens suddenly after a fracture or severe injury. It is a medical emergency.

Chronic Compartment Syndrome – happens gradually and immediately after repetitive exercise (Such as running or cycling). Not a medical emergency and can cause permanent damage.

Symptoms of Compartment Syndrome.
- Intense pain most common when the muscles are stretched.
- Tightness in the muscles.
- Tenderness in the affected area.
- Burning sensation or tingling.

What are the three mechanisms from which Compartment Syndrome occurs?
I. Trauma with a fracture.
II. Trauma without a fracture.
III. Non- traumatic fracture.

Non- traumatic causes of Compartment Syndrome include:
- Intramuscular hemorrhage.
- Nephrotic Syndrome.
- Intravenous Fluid extravasation

- Prolonged limb compression.
- Chronic exertional Compartment Syndrome.

What are the causes of Compartment Syndrome?
A. **Acute Compartment Syndrome** can be caused by
   - A broken bone or a crush injury- this is the most common cause.
   - A plaster cast or tight bandage being applied to the limb before it swells.
   - Burns.
   - Surgery to repair damaged or blocked blood vessels.
   - Sometimes without any obvious injury.
B. **Chronic Compartment Syndrome:** usually occurs in young people who do regular repetitive exercises, such as running or cycling. Caused by temporary swelling of the muscles during exercise affecting the blood supply to a whole group of muscles.

Treatments of Compartment Syndrome are:
- By surgical procedure called Emergency Fasciotomy.
- Can be relieved by stopping the exercise that triggers it and switch activities to a less strenuous activity.

Compression Stockings

How does Compression Stockings work?

Compression stockings gently squeeze your legs to move blood up your legs. This helps prevent legs swelling and to a lesser extent prevent blood clots.

If you have varicose veins, spider veins, or have just had surgery your doctor may prescribe compression stockings or anti-embolism stockings. It can be recommended for people who take long flights to keep blood from pooling in their legs. They can prevent scarring in the veins from forming blood clots. Compression stockings are not as effective as blood thinners in keeping clots from forming.

Confidentiality

According to NMC code "Confidentiality" states:
That every nurse must respect people's right to confidentiality and ensure they are informed on how and why information is shared to those who provide their care. In addition, it is a legal obligation and should be part of the terms and conditions of employment of any health professional.

Coronavirus

What is the virus called that causes coronavirus disease (covid-19)?

- Severe acute respiratory syndrome coronavirus 2(SARS-CoV-2)

What ate the symptoms of Covid-19?

- Fever or chills.
- Cough.
- Shortness of breath or difficulty breathing.
- Muscle or body aches.
- Headache.
- New loss of taste or smell.
- Sore throat.
- Congestion or running nose.
- Nausea or vomiting.
- Diarrhea.

When can one seek emergency medical attention?

- Trouble breathing.
- Persistent pain or preserve in the chest.
- Bluish lips or face.
- Inability to wake or stay awake.

What is the different between Influenza (flu) and COVID 19?

- They are contagious respiratory illnesses but are caused by different viruses.
- COVID 19 is speared by a virus named SARS- CoV-2) while flu is caused by a virus named Influenza Viruses.
- They share many characteristics.
- Testing can specifically identify of the diseases that is affecting the person.
  -

What is Coronavirus?

Coronaviruses are viruses which may cause respiratory infections (MERS-Middle East Respiration Syndrome and SARS Severe Acute Respiration Syndrome and COVID-19.

How does COVID -19 spread?

The disease spreads from person to person through small drop from the nose or mouth when a person infected with the virus coughs, sneezes and speaks. A non-infected person can be infected if they breathe in these droplets from an infected person with the virus. It can also be transmitted if this person touches any objects or surfaces, where the droplets land and then use the unwashed hand to touch the nose, eyes mouth. Hence, the needs to wash hands regularly with alcohol- base hand rub.

Can COVID – 19 be caught from a person who has no symptoms?

It is possible to be infected with COVID -19 from someone who has just had a mild cough and does not feel ill. People with no symptoms can transmit the virus.

How can we protect us from being infected?

(a) Practicing hand and respirators hygiene.

(b) Maintain at least one meter distance between yourself and other.

What do you do if you are in close contact with infected person?

- Stay at home (self-isolate).
- Monitor yourself for 14 days and avoid close contacts with others.
- If you develop difficulty in breathing, contact your healthcare provider immediately.
- Stay positive and keep In touch with loved ones.
- Do regular exercise at home.

How long does it take one to develop the symptoms after exposure to COVID 19?

It ranges from 1-14days. The period when the symptoms start manifesting majorly is from 5-6days.

What is the difference between self-Isolation, self–quarantine and Physical distancing?

- Self – isolation is separating people who are ill with the symptoms to prevent the spread of the disease.

- Self – quarantine is restricting activities or separating people who are not ill but may have been exposed to covid-19. This is to prevent the spread of the disease at the time when people just develop symptoms.

- Physical distancing means being physically apart from each other or others. Keep at least one metre distance from others.

Is there a treatment for COVID-19?

- Clinical trials are still going on according to World Health Organisation (WHO) in efforts to develop vaccine and medications to prevent and treat Covid-19.

The effective means for protection are:

- Wash your hands regularly.

- Avoiding touching your eyes, mouth and nose.

- Social and physical distance of at least one meter from others.

- Cover your cough, with the bend of elbow or, with tissue which you can easily dispose and then wash your hands properly for at least twenty seconds.

How do you properly wear a mask?

- Medical mask preferably recommended due to the minuet nature of the virus.

- Wash your hand or hand rub with a sanitizer.

- Place mask to your face and let the metal strip edge of the mask molds to the shape of your nose.

Consent

What is Consent to Treatment?

Consent to Treatment is the basic principle that a person must give permission before they receive any type of medical treatment, test or examination.

For consent to be valid, it must be voluntary and fully be informed, and the person consenting must have the capacity to make the decision.

How can Consent be given?

To get Consent means to:

- Get approval from the patient before the treatment or surgery commenced.
- Upholds people's right to be fully involved in decisions about their care.
- Respect and support people's right to accept or decline treatment of care.
- Be aware of the legislation regarding mental capacity.
- Be able to demonstrate that they have acted in someone's best interest if emergency care has been provided.
- It must be given voluntarily by a competent person who has been appropriately informed and who has the capacity to consent verbally or in writing for the intervention to be made.
- Someone could also give nonverbal consent as long as they understand the treatment or the diagnosis. E.g. holding out an arm for a blood test.
- To the health care professionals directly responsible for the person's current treatment, such as
- A nurse arranging for a blood test.
- A GP prescribing new medication.
- A surgeon planning an operation.
- The risks and benefits of the surgery which includes: disease process, diagnosis, nature of the surgery and prognosis. If treatment is withheld then alternative treatment option can be suggested.
- Informed consent must include:

- Patient's full name.
- Surgeon's name.

- Specific procedure.
- Signature of patient; next of kin or legal guardian.
- Witness (usually the nurse).
- Date.

The nurses' role involves that of advocacy and clarification of any misunderstanding. She should also support the patient's decision if he or she decides to withdraw the informed consent and refuse the procedure.

Advance Directives

Living Will: - Outlines the patient's wishes regarding medical treatment, life support and resuscitation measures.

Durable Power of Attorney: - Identifies the person who is authorized to make healthcare decision on the patient's behalf if the patient becomes incapacitated.

The preoperative nurse must be aware of the patient decision regarding advance directives. The preoperative nurse will document the patient's care and teachings giving during the preoperative phase, the document should be given to the nurse. The healthcare provider are required to inform their patient of their right and decisions making regarding healthcare choices. Advance directives also allow the individual to specify their preference of treatment, should they become unable to make in dependable health care decisions.

Conversion Disorder/Reaction

What are Conversion Disorder/ Reaction?

A Conversion disorder is a physical manifestation of emotions that displayed stressful event which result in defects in motor sensory function. Symptoms can be impaired balance, weakness in the extremity, paralysis. In an extremely loss of sensation, severe cases can cause deafness, seizures and blindness.

Extensive test done usually present normal, which ruled out medical disorders but the main fact, is that stressful condition are not pathologically based.

Associated Terms in Conversion Disorder:
- **Hypochondriasis** means strong fear of something.
- **Malingering** means faking illness.

Convert Administration

What is Convert Administration?
Convert administration is a situation where the patient medication is hidden in food or drink so that the patient would eventually take the medication without his knowledge. It is often practiced by health providers who knew that the outcome of such medication will give a positive result, but the patient would not comply if he or she knows.

For example, a patient whose blood pressure is too high needed some medication to bring it down. Having explained it to the patient concerned and the possible implications and the patient still refuses to give consent for the medication to be administered, then the healthcare provider decides to give the medication through food or drink without the knowledge of the patient.

This practice by some healthcare providers is unacceptable. If a patient refuses medications despite the explanations of the complications that may arise if such conditions are not treated with certain medications or procedure then as a nurse document and notify the Physician.

Crohn's Disease

What are the signs of Crohn's Diseases?
Crohn's disease is an inflammatory disease of the Intestine, majorly the Colon and ileum (the 3rd portion of the small Intestine). It is caused by bacterial, environmental, Immunological and genetic factors.

It occurs at any age and smokers are mostly at risk.

The signs:
1. Abdominal pain as a result of inflamed intestine.
2. It may cause ulcer which might lead to severe pain every time food passes through that part of the Intestine.
3. Cramps.
4. Frequent diarrhea.

5. Bloody stool.
6. Fever.

D

DATA

Data is a piece of information that can be measured and can be acceptable as factual.

Data Protection

Data Protection and Confidentiality

1. **Common law of Confidentiality**
   - Explicit consent.
   - Legal requirement.
   - Public interest.
2. **Human Right Act.**
   - Everyone has the right to have respect for his private life, his home and his correspondence.
3. **Data Protection.**
   - Data subject.

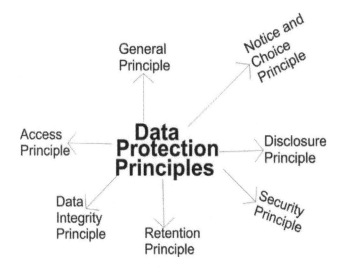

Dehydration

3 categories of Dehydration are?

1. Isotonic.
2. Hypertonic.
3. Hypotonic.

Signs and symptoms of Dehydration are?
- Thirst.
- Weight loss.
- Diseased urine output.
- Dry skin and muscles membrane.
- Fatigue.
- Increased body temperature.

Delegation

What is Delegation?
Delegation is the act of transferring authority to a competent individual to perform a selected task in a particular situation and the process of doing the work.

What are the Five Steps to Delegation?
1. Right task.
2. Right circumstance.
3. Right person.
4. Right direction /communication.
5. Right supervision

Delirium

Define Delirium?

Delirium is a distressing and serious disturbance underdiagnosed syndrome of acute attraction in mental state that results in confused thinking and reduced awareness of surroundings. It can be caused by intoxication or sleep deprivation. The causes aren't due to underlying disease condition.

Dementia Awareness

Define Dementia Awareness?

It describes the symptoms that occur when the brain is affected by certain diseases or conditions.

What is Dementia?

- It is an illness.
- It progresses gradually in which there is deterioration in cognitive functions.
- It is a brain damage.
- It is a loss of memory, language, problem solving and thinking abilities that can interfere with daily life activities.

Types of Dementia are?

1. Alzheimer disease- Is gradual and result as some part of the brain shrink.
2. Vascular dementia or emotional originated. It gets worst with time.
3. Lewy body dementia – falls, hallucination.
4. Mixed dementia.
5. Frontotemporal dementia
6. Mixed dementia. The most common combination is Alzheimer and vascular dementia.
7. Korsakoff syndrome- non progressive and alcohol related brain damage and alcohol abused. It is a type of dementia.

What are the symptoms of Dementia?
1. Memory losses
2. Learning difficulties
3. Language troubles
4. Difficulty in thinking
5. Bad decisions
6. Mood and personality changes
7. Loss of interest for some activities
8. Confusion
9. Cognitive problems associated with memory sometimes may contribute to the problem e.g. some drug interaction, drinking alcohol and thyroid problems.

Common issues with Dementia are:
- Not willing to go to the doctors.
- Getting lost.
- Losing important things.
- Make up stories.
- Refuses help sometimes.
- Can be rude.
- No solid sleep time.
- Neglect of personal care.
- Threatens Care givers.
- Unable to remember known faces or places visited to in the past.
- Undresses in public.
- Falls and injuries.
- Elopes and wanders
- Difficult to please.

What are the causes of dementia?
- Brain damage.
- Emotional distress.
- Depression.
- Cognitive challenges and illness.

Does the patient with dementia have the capacity to make decision?
Yes.

What is Depression?
Loss of pleasure or lack of interest in most activities, self-withdrawn, moody and melancholy disposition.

Diarrhea

What is diarrhea?
Diarrhea is loose watery and frequent bowel movement, usually last for few days. When it last for weeks, it could be a pathological problem.

Chronic causes of Diarrhea are:
- Crohn's disease
- Ulcerative colitis
- Malabsorption syndrome
- Irritable bowel syndrome.
- Lactose intolerance
- Chronic infections due bacteria, viruses or parasites infections.
- Some medications e.g. Antibiotics
- Gallbladder removal surgeries can cause it.

Differentiated Practice

What is Differentiated Practice?
Differentiated practice - Work is assigned according to different specialties in nursing. Examples: Neonatal nursing, Pediatrics nursing, ophthalmic nursing, preoperative nursing etc.

Discharge Planning

The Ten Steps for Discharge Planning are:
1. Start planning for discharge or transfer on admission.
2. Identify whether the patient has simple or complex discharge or transfer needs.
3. Develop a clinical management plan for every patient within 24hours of admission.

4. Co-ordinate the discharge and transfer, through effective leadership and handover responsibilities at ward level.
5. Set an expected date of discharge or transfers within 4 – 24hours of admission.
6. Review the clinical management plan with the patient each day, take necessary action and update progress toward the discharge or transfer date depending on what the condition may present or outcome.
7. Involve both patients and care giver so that they can make informed decision and a personalized care and then maximize their independence.
8. Plan discharge and transfer to take place within 7 days prior to discharge to deliver continuity of care to the patient.
9. Use a discharge checklist 24 - 48 hours before transfer.
10. Make decision to discharge and transfer patient each day.

Disclosure

What is Disclosure?
- A disclosure is when someone tells you directly they are being abused.
- You witness some events that led to the abuse or in the act e.g. suspicious bruising.
- Another professional, relatives or friends of the adult tells you about the abuse.
- You overheard someone voicing concerns about another person.

Responds to a Disclosure Do's
- Ensure immediate safety.
- Stay calm.
- Listen carefully and maintain eye contact.
- Reassure the adult and ensure they do the right thing.
- Explain your concerns to the adult.
- Request their concerns to make a report.
- Write down what you have seen or heard afterwards.
- Investigate with probing questions or prompt responses.
- Promise to keep secret
- Confront the abuser.

Don'ts

- Express shock, disgust or anger.
- Judge or conclude hastily.

Dosage Calculation

STANDARD FORMULA FOR CALCULATING A MEDICATION DOSAGE

D (desired) is the dosage that the health care provider prescribed.

A (available) is the dosage strength as stated on the medication label.

Q (quantity) is the volume or form in which the dosage strength is available such as tablets, capsules, or millilitres.

FORMULAS FOR INTRAVENOUS CALCULATION

Flow Rates

$$\frac{\text{Total volume X Drop factor}}{\text{Time in minutes}} = \text{Drops per minute}$$

Infusion Time

$$\frac{\text{Total volume to infuse}}{\text{millilitres per hour being infused}} = \text{Infusion time}$$

Numbers of millilitres per hour

$$\frac{\text{Total volume in millilitres}}{\text{Number of hours.}} = \text{Number of millilitres per hour.}$$

INFUSIONS PRESCRIBED BY UNIT DOSAGE PER HOUR

Calculation of these problems can be done using a 2- steps process.

1. Determine the amount of medication per 1 ml.
2. Determine the infusion rate or millilitres per hour.

Problem 1

Prescription: Continuous Heparin Sodium by IV at 1000 units per hour

Available: IV bag of 500mL D5w with 20,000 units of Heparin Sodium.

How many millilitres per hour are required to administer the correct dose?

Solution
Step1: Calculate the amount of medication (units) per millilitre (ml.).
Known amount of medication in solution
      Total volume of diluent

= Amount of medication per millilitre
20,000 units = 40 units/ 1 ml
   500ml

Step 2: Calculate millilitres per hour.

Dose per hour desired   = Infusion rate, or ml/hour
concentration per millilitre

1000 units =   **25 ml/hour**
  40 units

Problem 2:
**Prescription: Continuous Regular Insulin by IV at 10 units per hour
Available: IV bag of 100 ml NS with 50 units Regular Insulin.
How many millilitres per hour are required to administer the correct
dose?**

Solution
Step1: Calculate the amount of medication (units) per millilitre.

Known amount of medication in solution
Total volume of diluent
=Amount of medication per millilitre
50 units =   **0.5 units/ ml**
100ml

Step 2: Calculate millilitres per hour.
Dose per hour desired   = Infusion rate or ml/ hour
concentration per millilitres

10 units   =   **20ml/ hour.**
0.5 units/ml

PRACTICE QUESTIONS

1. A Physician's Order reads to administer an Intravenous (IV) dose of 400,000 units of Penicillin G Benzathine. The label on the 10ml ampoule sent from the pharmacy reads Penicillin G Benzathine 300,000 units/ml. The nurse prepares how many medications to administer the correct dose? Record your answer using one decimal place.

Solution
Using the medications dose formula:
Desired x M L = Millilitres per dose
 Available   1

400,000 units x I M L
   300,000 units   = Millilitres per dose
400,000
300,000 units = 1.33   =   **1.3ml**

2. A Physician's Order reads Phenytoin 0.2g orally twice daily. The medications label states that each capsule is 100mg. The nurse prepares how many capsule(s) to administer 1 dose?

Solution
Desired x capsule (s).
 Available   = Capsule (s) per dose
200mg x 1 capsule
   100mg   =   **2 Capsules.**

3. An Order was made of 1000ml of Normal Saline 0.9 percent to infuse over shows. The drop factor is 15 drops (gtt) 1ml.The nurse sets the flow rate of how many drops per minutes? Record your answer to the nearest whole number.

Solution

$$\frac{\text{Total volume x drop factor}}{\text{Time in minutes}} = \text{Drop per minute}$$

$$\frac{1000ml \times 15gtt}{480 \text{ minutes}} = \frac{15,000}{480} = 31.2, \text{ or}$$

$$= \quad \textbf{31gtt/min}$$

4. An Order was made of 1300 units /hour by continuous Intravenous (IV) Infusion. The Pharmacist prepares the medication and delivers an IV bag labelled repair in Sodium 200,000 units/250ml D_5W. An Infusion pump must be used to administer the medication. The nurse set the Infusion pump at how many millitre per hour to delivers 1300 units /hour? Answer should be recorded to the nearest whole.

Solution

$$\frac{\text{Known amount of medication in solution}}{\text{Total volume of diluent}}$$

= Amount of medication per millilitre

$$= \frac{20,000}{250ml} = \textbf{80 units ml}$$

Step 2.
Dose per hour desired = Infusion rate
Concentration per millitre

$$= \frac{1300 \text{ units}}{80 \text{ units /ml}} = \underline{16.25 \text{ or } 16\text{ml/hr.}}$$

5. **A Physician ordered 3000 ml of D_2W to be administered over a 24 hours period. The nurse determines how many millilitres per hour will be administered to the client?**

Solution
Use the intravenous (IV) formula to determine millilitres per hours.

I.e. $\frac{\text{Total volume in millilitres}}{\text{Numbers of hours}}$ = ML /hr.

: $\frac{3000\text{ml}}{24 \text{ hours}} = $ **125ml/hr.**

6. **An Order was made of 1000ml D_5W to Infuse at a rate of 125ml/hour. The nurse determines that it will take how many hours for 1 litre to infuse?**

Solution

$\frac{\text{Total volume to infuse}}{\text{Millilitres per hour being infused.}}$ = Infusion rate

$\frac{1000\text{mL}}{125\text{mL}} = $ **8 hours**

7. **An Order read Levothyroxine, 150mcg orally daily. The medication label reads Levothyroxine, 0.1mg/tablet. The nurse administers how many tablet(s) to the client?**

Solution

Desired x Tablet = Tablets per dose
Available

$$\frac{0.15mg}{0.1} \times tablets = \textbf{1.5 tablets.}$$

Dysphasia

It is difficulty in producing speech due to brain damage or disease. Aphasia is commonly used to describe both dysphasia and aphasia conditions and basically means loss, inability or difficulty in producing speech or language.

What is Dysphasia?

It is a language disorder marked by deficiency in generating of a speech and comprehension, ranging from no speech at all to difficulty naming certain objects. Both are learning disability and or a communicative disorder.

They have difficulty in talking, understanding, listening and writing and do numeric calculations.

E

Ectopic Pregnancy

Define Ectopic Pregnancy?

It is when a fertilized egg implants mostly on the fallopian tubes.

What are the symptoms of Ectopic Pregnancy?

Symptoms develop between the 4th to 12th weeks of pregnancy which are:

- Missed period.
- Vaginal bleeding.
- Tummy pain
- Pains at the pelvic or lower abdomen, mostly at the affected side.
- Abdominal cramps
- Nausea and vomiting
- Weakness and dizziness.
- Shoulder and neck pain, and could be at the rectum when going to the toilet.

End of Life Care

What is End of Life Care?

A component of palliative care has been defined as care that helps all those with advanced progressive, incurable conditions to live well as much as possible until death. It enables the supportive and palliative care needs of both patient and family to be identified and met throughout the last phase of life and into bereavement.

So therefore EOLC encompasses the holistic assessment and management of Physical care, Pain and other symptoms which includes; the provision of Psychological, Social, Financial, Spiritual and practical support for both the patient and their family care-givers in their place of choice, during the last years of life and includes cares given after bereavement.

The End Of Life Care Strategy – requires that an assessment is made of the patient's preferred place of care and how they wish to be cared for at the end of life.

Hospice is end of life care provided to a patient when the decision has been made that no further life – saving actions will be taken and when the provider has estimated that the patient has fewer than 6 months to live.

Enteral Feeding

What is Enteral Tube Feeding?

It refers to the delivery of nutritionally complete feed containing proteins, fats, carbohydrates, vitamins, mineral fluid and possibly dietary fibers directly into the gastrointestinal tract via a tube through the percutaneous route to the stomach, Jejunum or Duodenum.

What is an Enteral Feeding Tube? Enteral feeding tube allows liquid food to enter the stomach or intestine through a soft flexible tube.
- A gastrostomy (J- tube) is inserted in the stomach.
- A J-tube, (Jejunostomy tube) is inserted in the stomach but ends in the small intestine.

What are the indications for Enteral Tube Feeding?

Indications for enteral tube feeding:
- Depends on the active function of the GI tract.
- Cancer.
- Patient is unable to meet nutritional needs through oral intake alone.
- The gastrointestinal tract is not accessible and functioning well.
- Naos-gastric (NG tube) is inserted through the nose and down into the stomach, this is a type of tube feeding is for short term use.
- Nasojejunal (NJ – tube) is inserted through the nose down into the Jejunal, the second part of the small intestine.
- It is anticipated that this function will meet all nutritional needs.

Types of Enteral Feeding
  a. Nasogastric.
  b. Nasoduodenal.
  c. Nasojejunal.

Different types of Feeding Tube
  1. Naso- gastric (Na) Tube.
  2. Naso jejunal Tube.
  3. Gastrostomy Tube.
  4. Jejunostomy Tube.

The test precision for Enteral Tube placement is?
The surest test is the X-ray and PH value which is about 7.4.

Equality and Diversity

Equality: is ensuring individuals or groups are treated fairly, in order to promote a fair equal treatment to the society. Everyone should have an equal opportunity regardless of their Race, Gender, Disability, Religion, Age, and Sex Orientation. Equality is not about being politically correct or telling people what they can and can't say, it's about treating others as you would want to be treated.

Diversity: is about recognizing individuals as well as group differences and placing a positive value on diversity. Diversity is everything that is different about everybody. The meanings are:
  • D –Different.
  • I –Individuals.
  • V –Value.
  • E –Each other.
  • R –Regular.
  • S –Skin.
  • I –Intellect.
  • T –Talent or.
  • Y –Years.

Diversity is a set of conscious practices that is more than just acknowledging and or tolerating differences of others.

Eye Administration Medication

What are the steps for proper eye administration instillation?

1. Wash your hands properly with soap and water.
2. Remove glasses and or Contact lenses.
3. Shake the container for 10 seconds, if instructed by the Physician or Pharmacist.
4. Remove the cap from the medication bottle and ensure that it does not touch the tip of the container.
5. Let the patient tilt the head backward in a fowler's or supine position.
6. Pull the lower eye down against the cheek (Conjunctiva).
7. Instruct the patient to look up.
8. Squeeze a drop in the Conjunctiva sac.
9. Ask the patient to close the eye for a few minutes.
10. Wait 3 to 5 minutes before applying another drop.
11. Do not let the medication bottle touch the eyeball.

F

Functional method

What is Functional Method?

It is task- oriented, whereby a particular nursing function is assigned to each staff member, medication nurse, Pediatric nurse, wound dressing nurse. These are examples of this method.

Fundamental Values

The NMC"6" C Values are;

1. Compassion.
2. Competence.
3. Communication.
4. Courage.
5. Commitment.
6. Care

G

Gillick Competent

Gillick Competent means that: Whatever reason a particular decision is needed, a young person who is younger than eighteen years old who:

- Understands the risks & benefits of treatments.
- Understands the problem of his health and its implications.
- Understands the consequences if not treated.
- Understands the alternative options narrated to him.
- Understands the Implications on the family.
- Is able to retain and recall the information.
- Is able to determine the benefits and or the disadvantages.
- Is able to make and communicate reasonable and good decisions regarding their wishes.

Such a young person can give consent to treatment regarding his condition and this is known as **Gillick Competent.**

If a young person who is Gillick competent, ask professionals not to share information about their treatment, their wishes can be honoured, unless where there are safety issues and the information is required to be shared.

Young persons under eighteen years old who are regarded as Gillick competent can make decisions regarding their treatment and can give consent to treatment, even though their parents are not in agreement.

It does however often benefit the child and the family if the child is supported in his/her decisions regarding treatment by the family.

Glomerulonephritis

Define Glomerulonephritis:

It is an infection and inflammation of the Glomeruli.

What are the Symptoms of Glomerulonephritis?

- Haematuria.
- Frothy urine.
- Leg oedema.
- Weakness.
- Joint pains.

It can be predisposed by high blood pressure or respiratory disorder.

Causes of Glomerulonephritis
- Systemic Lupus Erythematous or vacuities.
- Hepatitis B or C.
- HIV.

The treatments for Glomerulonephritis are:
- Low salt diet.
- ACE inhibitors medications to help, protect the kidney.

List the complications of Glomerulonephritis:
- High blood pressure.
- High cholesterol.
- Blood clots (deep vein thrombosis or pulmonary embolism).
- Chronic kidney disease.
- Kidney failure.

H
Hashimotos Disease

What are the symptoms of Hashimoto's Disease?
Hashimoto's Disease is also known as Hypothyroidism. Normal thyroid help to produce energy, skin hydration, thermostat for normal body temperature and energy balance. If the thyroid is diseased with low secretion of thyroid hormone, then the symptoms present are as follows:
- Fatigue & weakness.
- Dry skin.
- Cold due to decrease thermostat.
- Weight gain.

Holistic Care

What is Holistic Care?

A system of comprehensive or total patient care that consider the physical, emotional, social, economic and spiritual needs of the person; his or her response to illness, the effect of the illness and the ability to meet self-care needs.

Holistic nurses develop therapy partnerships with others to strengthen their response and promote healing and wholeness (Dossey Keagan, 2016).

FIVE CORE VALUES OF HOLISTIC NURSING PRACTICE.

- Holistic philosophy, theory and ethics.
- Holistic caring process.
- Holistic communication, therapeutic healing, environmental and cultural competence.
- Holistic education and research.

HOLISTIC CARING PROCESS

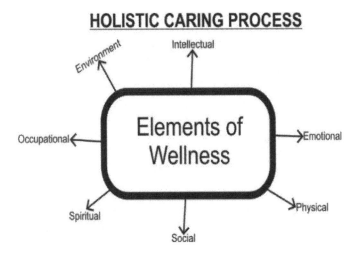

Hydrocolloid

What is Hydrocolloid?

A hydrocolloid dressing is water based transparent type of dressing for wounds. It provides an insulating moist and m healing environment that protects wounds that is not infected. In the process of healing it allows the body own enzyme to take in the healing. Its advantage is that it is easily applied and it does not need to be changed often. It is indicated for superficial wounds with low drainage. While hydrocolloid patches gently absorbs excess fluids, oils, pus from pimples.

Hydrostatic Pressure

What is Hydrostatic Pressure?

Itis caused by the pumping action of the heart and the resistances of blood vessel at the arteriole end of the capillary.

Differences and Similarities

Hydrostatic pressure exceeds **Osmotic pressure** by moving solutes out of the plasma and into interstitial space.

While at the venous the hydrostatic **pressure is reduced** and the **osmotic pressure within the vessel** (plasma) is higher, so water is pulled back into the vessel and circulatory volume.

I

Infectious Prevention &Control

What is Universal Precaution?

These are precautions that are taken with blood and "high-risk" body fluids. They are based on the principles that any individual can be affected with a blood borne virus such as HIV or hepatitis B and so pose a risk of infectious on the individual. This practice can be regarded as completely "Risk free".

What is Standard Precaution?

It is the action that should be taken in every care situation to protect patient and others from infections regardless of what is known of the patient status in respect to infection. This includes:

- Hand hygiene at every moments, including before and after each patient contacts.
- Care in the use and disposal of sharps.
- The correct use of personal protective equipment for contact with all blood, body fluids, secretions and excretions.
- Providing care in a suitably clean environment with adequate decontaminated equipment.
- The safe disposal of waste.
- The safe management of used linen.

Another term for Standard Precaution is:
Universal Precaution or Standard Precautions or Biosafety Precaution.

Precaution Standard applies to
- Blood.
- Body fluid with visible blood.
- Genital secretion.
- Cerebro spinal fluid (CSF).
- Pleural / Peritoneal / Pericardia fluid.
- Synovial / amniotic fluids.
- Breast milk.

Transmission-based Precautions are classified into;
- Contact precaution.
- Enteric precaution.
- Droplet precaution.
- Air borne precaution.

Causes of infection are;
- Bacteria.
- Fungi.
- Viruses.
- Protozoa.
- Prions.
- Helminths.
- Arthropods.
- Lice, scabies.

The Modes of Transmission are;
- Direct contact.
- Droplet transmission.
- Airborne transmission.
- Parental transmission.
- Vector transmission.
- Faecal – oral transmission.

Which action is necessary to maintain asepsis during a sterile dressing change?
After scrubbing for the procedure, hold your elbows close to your body.

Personal Protective Equipment (PPE)
- Sterile gloves.
- Eye protection (Eye Goggle, Face shield)
- Mask
- Foot protection (booth)
- Disposable gloves.
- Disposable aprons.

What is the correct order and steps for the nurse to remove the PPE after caring for a patient in isolation as well as order contagious procedure?
i.   Gloves are to be removed by extension of the arms and slowly peel one glove downward, turning it inside out. With the ungloved hand, slide a finger under the inside portion of the remaining glove, turning inside out and discard.
ii. Remove Goggles/Face shield by grasping the ear pieces or headband.
iii. Remove gown after unfastening the neck and the waist then pull gown forward away from the body.
iv. Mask is removed by only touching the ties but the front of the mask is not touched.

Aseptic Technique

Aseptic Technique is the practice of carrying out a procedure in such a way that you minimize the risk of introducing contamination into a vulnerable area or contaminating invasive devices.

Few examples of aseptic procedures are;
- Surgical joint replacement.
- Urine catheterization.
- Peripheral intravenous connection.
- Change of wound dressing.

Infections Identified and Their Respective Mode of Transmission.

INFECTIONS	MODE OF TRANSMISSION
Measles. Meningococcal.	Droplet/faecal oral.
Septicaemia.	Droplet.
MRSA.	Contact/droplet.
Mungs.	Droplets.
No virus / small round structured virus (SRSV).	Faecal/oral contact.
Rota virus.	Droplet/faecal/oral.
Rubella.	Droplet.
Salmonella or shigella.	Faecal- oral.
) Scabies.	Contact.
) Scarlet fever.	Droplet.
) Severe acute respiratory syndrome.	Droplet/contact.
) Shingles (herpes zoster).	Contact.
) Tuberculosis.	Contact/airborne.
) Typhoid fever.	Faecal – oral.
) Escherichia coli (E.coli).	Faecal – oral.
) Viral hemorrhage fever.	Droplet/blood/contact.

) Lassa fever.	Droplet/blood/contact.
) Ebola.	Droplet/blood/contact.
) COVID 19 or Corona Virus	Droplet/ airborne/contact
) HIV/AIDS	Blood Contact/Secretion

Infusion Administration

What is the cause of excessive IV fluid administration?
Increased Circulatory volumes as a result of electrolytes imbalance or over balance, administration of overload of fluids within a short period of time, renal and cardiovascular conditions, age factor, type of medications administered.

Intelligent Kindness

Intelligent Kindness means - Compassion, care given through professional relationship based on Empathy, Respect and Dignity.

K

Kidney Infection

What is a Kidney Infection? A Kidney Infection is a type of urinary tract infection which is caused by bacteria called Escherichia Coli (E Coli).This bacteria moves from the genitals through the urethra into the bladder and up the ureters which connect the bladder to the kidneys.

What are the symptoms of Kidney Infection?

- Strong urge to urinate
- Fever
- Frequent urination.
- Burning sensation when urinating.
- Cloudy urine and foul smelling urine.
- Abdominal pain

- Groin pain, flank, back and side pains.
- Haematuria.

How can Kidney Infection be prevented?
- Drinking plenty of fluid.
- Urinating as soon as you feel the urge.
- Washing the genitals daily.
- Treating constipation.
- Females wiping from front to backward after urinating.
- Urinating after sex.
- Not using condoms or diaphragm that has been coated with spermicide if you are prone to getting UTI's.

Korotkoff

What is Korotkoff?

In measuring the blood pressure, a stethoscope is placed over the heart that has been anchored by inflated blood pressure cuff, as you slowly deflect the cuff the sounds produced. The series of sounds that you hear through the stethoscope are Korotkoff.

What are the sounds produced?

The sounds produced are based on the phases of sound during the process. The first sound heard as soon as the cuff is slowly deflated is tapping sound, followed by swishing, knocking, muffling and finally the point at which all sounds finally disappear completely is the diastolic pressure.

The systolic blood pressure is taken as the first Korotkoff sound and the diastolic blood pressure is the fifth Korotkoff sound, it is barely audible. Recent studies have moved the use of the fifth Korotkoff sound (i.e. silence) as the diastolic blood pressure.

1. Tapping sound.
2. Swishing sound.
3. Knocking sound

4.   Muffling sound.

5.   Silence as the diastolic blood pressure stop.

L

Laboratory Diagnostics

LABORATORY TESTS	BODY PARTS
Barium Enema	Lower GI series identifies Inflammation, tumours structure, varies, and inguinal hernia
Cholecystography	Gall bladder series; ingestion of iodine before the procedure, it identifies stones in the gallbladder of the bile duct and tumors or other obstructions.
Cholangiography	Dye is injected into the bile duct and pancreatic duct through endoscopic tube then visualise with radiology to determine potency of ducts from liver and gall bladder. Also done are E R C P – Endoscopic retrograde Cholangio Pancreatrography.
Radionuclide Imaging	Detects lesions of the liver or pancreas.
Computed Tomography (CT)	Use for structures that may not be seen otherwise, NPO for 6-8 hours prior test.
Magnetic Resonance Imaging(MRI)	To visualize structures contrast used. N P O 6-8hours prior to test.
Ultrasonography	Shows size and location of Organs. Detect Cholecystitis, Cholelithiasis, Pyloric stenosis waves are directed.
Percutaneous liver biopsy	A needle is placed through the abdominal wall to obtain small amount of liver tissue. (PT, I N R, PTT) coagulation

	studies.
Liver Biopsy	Assist client to roll to right side after procedure. Avoid cough, straining, lifting or strenuous activity.
GI Endoscopy, Colonoscopy EGO – Esophagogastroduodenoscopy	Direct visualisation, dietary, Fluid restriction. Asses gag reflex before any oral intake.
Stool Analysis	Detect RBC's, WBC's, fat, bacteria or parasites.
The Labs	-CBC- (RBC, WBC). -Urinalysis. -Serum bilirubin. -Cholesterol (lipids- may show Mal absorption). -Prothrombin time (PT). -Amylase. -Lipase.
Gastric Analysis	-Analyses of gastric mucosa. - Analyses of gastric retention in client with pyloric or duodenal obstruction. -Client is on NPO 8-12hours prior to the procedure. -Gastric contents are aspirated through NG tube 15 minutes to 1hour, and PH and cytology performed.
Helicobacter Pyloric Test, P Y test	-Detects H. Pyloric (bacteria associated with peptic ulcers) (a). Transmitted person to person, oral-faecal, oral-oral. (b). Bores through mucous lining of the stomach and invades it. (c). Causes damage and allows stomach acid to penetrate tissue.

Laceration

How can you describe Laceration?

Lacerations are caused by a blunt force, tearing tissues or cut in the skin. They commonly occur as a result of a fall. In approximated wound, edges are not defined.

Lateral Positioning

What are the indications for positioning a patient laterally?

The indications for positioning the patient side-lying (Lateral) are:

- Compromised venous return provide abdominal mass. So keeping a patient in this position ease comfort and to enable adequate circulation.
- Pregnancy to relieve pressure on the diaphragm and heart.
- Cancer to ease comfort and have proper alignment of the body and to relieve pain.
- Surgery to prevent complications and ease pain.

Leadership in Nursing

What is Leadership?

Leadership is the ability to define a vision and guide individuals and groups toward that vision while maintaining group momentum through promoting teamwork effectiveness and then lead by example.

Who is a Nurse Leader?

A nurse leader is that nurse who identifies opportunities for improvement and volunteers to inspire other having the initiative to achieve a common goal. Develop treatment plan, implement and evaluate treatment results and manage patients-nursing team. The nurse leader has two major qualities; they are excellent clinicians (b) He or she mentors and have informal opinion which guides their subordinates.

What are the qualities of a Leader in Nursing?
 a. Caring.
 b. Empathy.
 c. Eagerness to learn.
 d. Organizational skill.
 e. Interpersonal skill.
 f. Self-awareness.

 g. Confident
 h. Ability to co-ordinate and motivates.

What are the Nursing Leadership Styles?
 a. Democratic leadership.
 b. Autocratic leadership.
 c. Transformation leadership.
 d. Laissez faire leadership.

Case Management - the nurse is responsible for total patient care during her shift.
Primary Nursing – the nurse cares for her primary patient's or the same patient every time she works and for as long as the patient remains in her unit.

Learning Disability
What is Learning Disability?

A learning disability is a way a person understand information and communicates. It means having difficulty to understand new and complex information, difficulty to learn new skills and to cope independently.

What are the types of learning disability? This is classified into:

 (a) Mild. (b) Moderate. (c) And Severe.

What are the causes of learning disability?

It means that the person brain development is affected at birth or at infancy due to:

a. Maternal illness.
b. Fetal distress.
c. Gene mutation.
d. Genetically abnormalities
e. Illness at infancy.

It could be due to brain injury in early childhood which resulted to:

- Cerebral.
- Autism.
- Epilepsy.

Signs of learning disability

- Difficulty with attention.
- Longer time to complete tasks.
- Needs repeated direction.
- Difficulty in organising activities.
- Poor reading comprehension.
- Poor memory.
- Avoid assignments.
- Easily frustrated with school activities and have low self-esteem.

Liver Biopsy

What is the immediate management after Liver Biopsy?

Immediately after the biopsy;

- Pressure is applied at biopsy site to prevent bleeding.
- Bandage is placed on the Incision.
- The patient is to lie on the right side for at least one hour following the procedure and then additional 3 hours after the first one hour.
- Blood pressure and heart rate is regularly monitored.
- It is an outpatient procedure.

Lumbar Positioning

a. To position the patient during the procedure of Lumbar puncture is to assist the patient positioned to the lateral (side lying), with the back bowed at the edge of the examining table, the knees flexed up to the abdomen, and the neck flexed so that the chin is resting on the chest.

b. After the procedure, place the client in the supine position for 4 to 12 hours as prescribed.

M

Manual Handling

What is Manual Handling?

Manual handling means any activity requiring the use of force exerted by a person to lift, lower, push, hold or carry, or otherwise move, hold or restrain a person, animal or thing.

In manual handling, weight bearing will be affected by:

- Pain.
- Weakness.
- Sensory changes
- Confidence.

What are the techniques of moving and handling a patient?

1. Align in good posture.
2. Keep knees bent with feet wide apart.
3. Distribute weight evenly over both legs and keep shoulders straight and centred over hips.
4. Keep stomach muscles tight and buttocks tucked under, while your head is up and at the chin's level.
5. Balance and stability should be achieved.
6. Keep a wide base and low centres of gravity.
7. Spread your legs, bend your knees and lower your torso to remain stable on your feet.

In handling of an unconsciousness patient manually, what are you expected to do?

Unconsciousness means a physiological state in which the patient is unresponsive to sensory stimuli and lack awareness of self and the environment (Hickey 2000).

In manual handling of a patient in this condition needs extreme care. The body alignment has to be centrally placed on the bed. There is the need for changing the positions two hourly to avoid pressure sore. Observe and monitor closely.

Effects of immobility on Unconscious patients. Respiratory complications such as Atelectasis, Pneumonia, Aspiration and Airway Obstruction and then the muscles will atrophy and decreased muscle strength.

- Deep vein thrombosis and pulmonary embolism
- In the process of immobility, DVT is increased on patients. This is due to factors such as blood pooling in the legs, hypercoagulability and prolonged pressure from immobility in bed.
- **For the amputee patient below knee extension;**
  Maintain knee extension in bed, to prevent knee flexion contracture. While seated in the chair, support knee point and prevent excursion of knee flexion.
- **For above, the knee amputee:** Maintain hip in a neutral position, to maintain hip extension and to prevent excessive hip flexion.

Medicine Management

What is Medicine Management?

Medicine Management involves doing one or all of the following:

a. Deciding which medicines to give.
b. Selecting which medicines to give.
c. Measuring out liquid medicines.
d. Apply appropriate cream, ointment or drops for treatment.
e. Giving a person medicine to swallow, apply or inhale.

Safety Tips for Medicine Management are as follows:
1. Check the date making sure it has not expired.
2. Carry a list of all your medicines and keep it up to date. Make sure the list matches with the actual medicines.
3. Keep medicines bottle together.
4. Keep a particular type of pill in each bottle. Just in case you don't know what the pills are for.
5. Use a medicine box; this helps you to know the days and times of taken the medicines.
6. Allow enough time to get your medications refilled, do not wait for the last pill before you get the refill. Give at least one week notice.
7. Be careful of the medicine name due to the generic or brand name could be different.
8. Be careful of drug interactions, some drugs should not be taken with other types of medications. Check the prescription list to know when to take the medication and if it should be taken with food, fluid or a suspension.
9. Be careful, observe for side effects, call the doctor and follow the doctor's instructions if affected.

Medication Management

Medication is a substance use for medical transformation, especially meant for therapeutic purposes. E.g. Medicines or medications, herbals etc.

The side effects of some medications are?
Examples:

NSAIDS- Bleeding /Ulcers...

Anticoagulants – Bleeding.

Benadryl –Drowsiness.

Antibiotic – Diarrhea.

Allergic reaction and side effect leads to Adverse Drug Reaction (ADR).

Narcotic and Antidepressant user in the elderly leads to a greater risk for fall.

Common drug interaction examples include:
1. Aspirin and Warfarin (Coumadin).
2. Antacids and certain Antibiotics.
3. Ginkgo Biloba and Warfarin (Coumadin).

Common drug food interaction
1. Calcium rich in dairy products, antacids, and vitamins containing iron can all decrease the effects of antibiotics especially Tetracycline.
2. Grapefruit juice can inhibit enzymes in the liver which involved in drug metabolism, and there by increasing the effect of this medication on the patients.
3. Foods high in Vitamin K (green leafy vegetables) and others decrease the effectiveness of Coumadin.

What can you do to avoid drug interaction?
1. Read the labels of all your medications carefully.
2. Know the benefits and potentials risk of all your medications.
3. Talk to your doctor or pharmacist before taken any new medication.
4. Keep the accurate list of all the medications you administer including dosages and frequency of prescription.
5. Ensure the source is genuine if you are a home nurse care giver.
6. Keep medications in original prescription bottles.

Mental Capacity Act

What is Mental Capacity Act (MCA)?
MCA can help protect and empower one to make their own decisions about their care and treatment if they lack mental capacity.

Mental Capacity Act Codes are;
Presume that a person has mental capacity until they are:
- Unable to understand information given to them to make choices.
- Can understand but are unable to retain information.

- Are unable to weigh up and relate the information accurately to their situation.
- Are unable to communicate their wishes or choices by any means.

With these factors in place MCA recommends that determining an individual's decision making capacity is best achieved through Multidisciplinary Assessment.

Methicillin Resistant Staphylococcus Aureus
Define MRSA?
Methicillin Resistant Staphylococcus Aureus is the most common kind of bacteria often found in hospitals with patients admitted in the wards. They get into the body through burns, urinary catheters etc.

What are the symptoms of MRSA?
a. Redness,
b. Swelling,
c. Warmth,
d. Pains,
e. Pus.

Later signs includes:
1. High temperature of $38^{0c.}$
2. Chills.
3. Dizziness.
4. Confusion.

What are the Treatments?
a. Apply antibacterial shampoo.
b. Change your towels, clothes and bed lines daily during treatment. Laundry or washed separately from other patient's clothes and at a high temperature.

N

Nasogastric Tube

What are the steps in a chronological order for placing a nasogastric tube in a client?

i. Explain procedure to the client and assist client to high fowler's position if possible.
ii. Measure the tubing from the tip of the nose to the tip of the ear lobe and to the tip of the xiphoid then mark it with adhesive tape.
iii. Put on your gloves and lubricate the tip.
iv. Gradually insert the tube and when tubing reaches the mark, anchor the tube using tape.
v. Aspirate gently to collect gastric contents and test PH.

What are the chronological orders for removing a nasogastric tube from a patient?

i. Assess bowel function by auscultation for peristalsis.
ii. Assist client into semi Fowler's position.
iii. Flush tube with 10 ml of normal saline. Flushing usually ensures that the tube doesn't contain stomach contents that could irritate tissues during tube removal.
iv. Ask client to hold her breath. This is to close epiglottis.
v. Withdraw the tube gently and steadily.

List the clinical findings the nurse should monitor for with a client who has a nasogastric tube with suctioning?

The clinical findings are related to hypokalemia and hyponatremia. These are Flat T waves on ECG, muscle weakness, nausea, fatigue, and muscle cramps in the case of hypokalemia while the hyponatremia may present with tachycardia, headache, anorexia, lethargy, hypotension, confusion, hypo bowel sounds, muscle weakness, seizures and coma.

Needle Stick Injury

What actions would u take in the case of a Needle Stick Injury?

I.   Wash the affected body parts with soap and water.

II.   Disinfect area with an alcohol swab.

III.   Apply a sterile dressing if necessary.

IV.   Go to the closest hospital emergency room for assessment as soon as possible within 2 hours of the occurrence. Ensure that you receive the needle stick exposure package and get tested for HIV at once, then 6 weeks, 6 months and a year later.

V.   Inform the manager or supervisor on how the injury occurred.

VI.   Report the incident.

VII.   Accurately filled up the incident report form and return to your manager.

NOROVIRUS

Norovirus causes diarrhea and vomiting, is one of the most common stomach problems. It is also called the Winter Vomiting Bug because it is more common in winter, it can be transmitted any time of the year. Norovirus can be very unpleasant but it usually clears up by itself in a few days.

Symptoms of Norovirus
- Suddenly feeling sick.
- Projectile vomiting.
- Diarrhea
- Fever.
- Headaches
- Stomach cramps.
- Aching limbs.

The symptoms appear one to two days after being infected and last up to 2 or 3 days.

What do you do when infected by Norovirus?

- Drink plenty of fluids.
- Take **analgesics** for any fever or aches and pain.
- Get plenty of rest.
- Eat a balanced meal.
- Take prepared rehydration solutions if you have signs of dehydration, for example, dark urine.
- Take Antidiarrheal and Anti-emetic (anti-vomiting) medications.

Norovirus can spread very easily, **wash your hands** regularly. Usually antibiotics do not help because it is also caused by a virus.

Consult a doctor if:
- A baby or child has passed 6 or more watery stools in the past 24 hours, or has vomited 3 times or more in the past 24 hours.
- A baby or child is less responsive, feverish, or has pale skin.
- A patient is dehydrated, dizzy, and could not pass urine or passes small amount of urine or reduced consciousness.
- Babies and elderly people who have a greater risk of becoming dehydrated.
- Bloody diarrhea.
- If symptoms haven't started to improve after a few days.

How does Norovirus spread?
Norovirus spreads very easily in public places such as hospitals, nursing homes and schools. Easily transmissible through small particles of vomit or faces from an infected person and get into your mouth, through:

- Close contact with someone with norovirus – they may breathe out small particles containing the virus that you could inhale.
- Touching contaminated surfaces or objects – the virus can survive outside the body for several days.
- Eating contaminated food – this can happen if an infected person doesn't wash their hands before handling food.

A person with norovirus is most infectious from when their symptoms start until 48 hours after all their symptoms have passed, although they may also be infectious for a short time before and after this. One can get norovirus more than once because the virus is always changing, so your body is unable to build up long-term resistance to it.

How can one prevent Norovirus?
It's not always possible to avoid getting norovirus, but the steps below can help stop the virus from spreading:

- Stay off work or school until at least 48 hours after the symptoms have passed.
- You should also avoid visiting anyone in hospital during this time.
- **Thoroughly wash your hands** frequently with soap and water.
- Disinfect any surface or object that could be contaminated.
- Wash any item of clothing or bedding that could have become contaminated separately, on a hot water to ensure the virus is killed.

- Don't share towels and flannels.
- Flush away any infected faces or vomitus in the toilet and clean the surrounding area with disinfectant.
- Avoid eating raw, unwashed produce and only eat oysters from a reliable source, as oysters can carry norovirus.

Nursing and Midwifery Council (NMC) Codes

Prioritise people

You put the interests of people using or needing nursing or midwifery services first. You make their care and safety your main concern and make sure that their dignity is preserved and their needs are recognised, assessed and responded to. You make sure that those receiving care are treated with respect, that their rights are upheld and that any discriminatory attitudes and behaviours towards those receiving care are challenged.

1. Treat people as individuals and uphold their dignity.

To achieve this, you must:

1.1 Treat people with kindness, respect and compassion.

1.2 Make sure you deliver the fundamentals of care effectively.

1.3 Avoid making assumptions and recognise diversity and individual choice.

1.4 Make sure that any treatment, assistance or care for which you are responsible for is delivered without undue delay.

1.5 Respect and uphold people's human rights.

2. Listen to people and respond to their preferences and concerns.

To achieve this, you must:

2.1 Work in partnership with people to make sure you deliver care effectively.

2.2 Recognise and respect the contribution that people can make to their own health and wellbeing.

2.3 Encourage and empower people to share decisions about their treatment and care.

2.4 Respect the level to which people receiving care want to be involved in decisions about their own health, wellbeing and care.

2.5 Respect, support and document a person's right to accept or refuse care and treatment.

2.6 Recognise when people are anxious or in distress and respond compassionately and politely.

The fundamentals of care include, but are not limited to, nutrition, hydration, bladder and bowel care, physical handling and making sure that those receiving care are kept in clean and hygienic conditions.

It includes making sure that those receiving care have adequate access to nutrition and hydration, and making sure that you provide help to those who are not able to feed themselves or drink fluid unaided.

3. Make sure that people's physical, social and psychological needs are assessed and responded to.

To achieve this, you must:

3.1 Pay special attention to promoting wellbeing, preventing ill health and meeting the changing health and care needs of people during all life stages.

3.2 Recognise and respond compassionately to the needs of those who are in the last few days and hours of life.

3.3 Act in partnership with those receiving care, helping them to access relevant health and social care, information and support when they need it, and;.

3.4 Act as an advocate for the vulnerable, challenging poor practice and discriminatory attitudes and behaviour relating to their care.

4. Act in the best interests of people at all times.

To achieve this, you must:

4.1 Balance the need to act in the best interests of people at all times with the requirement to respect a person's right to accept or refuse treatment.

4.2 Make sure that you get properly informed consent and document it before carrying out any action.

4.3 Keep to all relevant laws about mental capacity that apply in the country in which you are practicing, and make sure that the rights and best interests of those who lack capacity are still at the centre of the decision-making process.

4.4 Tell colleagues, your manager and the person receiving care if you have a conscientious objection to a particular procedure and arrange for a suitably qualified colleague to take over responsibility for that person's care (see the note below).

5. Respect people's right to privacy and confidentiality.

As a nurse or midwife, you owe a duty of confidentiality to all those who are receiving care. This includes making sure that they are informed about their care and that information about them is shared appropriately.

To achieve this, you must:

5.1 Respect a person's right to privacy in all aspects of their care.

5.2 Make sure that people are informed about how and why information is used and shared by those who will be providing care.

5.3 Respect that a person's right to privacy and confidentiality continues after they have died.

5.4 Share necessary information with other healthcare professionals and agencies only when the interests of patient safety and public protection override the need for confidentiality, and.

5.5 Share with people, their families and their carers, as far as the law allows, the information they want or need to know about their health, care and ongoing treatment sensitively and in a way they can understand.

Please visit: **www.nmc.org.uk/standards**

Practice effectively

You assess need and deliver or advice on treatment, or give help (including preventative or rehabilitative care) without too much delay and to the best of your abilities, on the basis of the best evidence available and best practice. You communicate effectively, keeping clear and accurate records and sharing skills, knowledge and experience where appropriate. You reflect and act on any feedback you receive to improve your practice.

6. Always practice in line with the best available evidence.

To achieve this, you must:

6.1 Make sure that any information or advice given is evidence-based, including information relating to using any healthcare products or services, and.

6.2 Maintain the knowledge and skills you need for safe and effective practice.

7. Communicate clearly

To achieve this, you must:

7.1 Use terms that people in your care, colleagues and the public can understand.

7.2 Take reasonable steps to meet people's language and communication needs, providing, wherever possible, assistance to those who need help to communicate their own or other people's needs.

7.3 Use a range of verbal and non-verbal communication methods, and consider cultural sensitivities, to better understand and respond to people's personal and health needs.

7.4 Check people's understanding from time to time to keep misunderstanding or mistakes to a minimum, and.

7.5 Be able to communicate clearly and effectively in English.

8. Work cooperatively

To achieve this, you must:

8.1 Respect the skills, expertise and contributions of your colleagues, referring matters to them when appropriate.

8.2 Maintain effective communication with colleagues.

8.3 Keep colleagues informed when you are sharing the care of individuals with other healthcare professionals and staff.

8.4 Work with colleagues to evaluate the quality of your work and that of the team.

8.5 Work with colleagues to preserve the safety of those receiving care.

8.6 Share information to identify and reduce risk.

8.7 Be supportive of colleagues who are encountering health or performance problems. However, this support must never compromise or be at the expense of patient or public safety.

9. Share your skills, knowledge and experience for the benefit of people receiving care and your colleagues.

To achieve this, you must:

9.1 Provide honest, accurate and constructive feedback to colleagues.

9.2 Gather and reflect on feedback from a variety of sources, using it to improve your practice and performance.

9.3 Deal with differences of professional opinion with colleagues by discussion and informed debate, respecting their views and opinions and behaving in a professional way at all times, and.

9.4 Support students' and colleagues' learning to help them develop their professional competence and confidence.

10. Keep clear and accurate records relevant to your practice.

This includes but is not limited to patient records. It includes all records that are relevant to your scope of practice.

To achieve this, you must:

10.1 Complete all records at the time or as soon as possible after an event, recording if the notes are written sometime after the event.

10.2 Identify any risks or problems that have arisen and the steps taken to deal with them, so that colleagues who use the records have all the information they need.

10.3 Complete all records accurately and without any falsification, taking immediate and appropriate action if you become aware that someone has not kept to these requirements.

10.4 Attribute any entries you make in any paper or electronic records to youself, making sure they are clearly written, dated and timed, and do not include unnecessary abbreviations, jargon or speculation.

10.5 Take all steps to make sure that all records are kept securely.

10.6 Collect, treat and store all data and research findings appropriately.

11 Be accountable for your decisions to delegate tasks and duties to other people.

To achieve this, you must:

11.1 Only delegate tasks and duties that are within the other person's scope of competence, making sure that they fully understand your instructions.

11.2 Make sure that everyone you delegate tasks to is adequately supervised and supported so they can provide safe and compassionate care, and

11.3 Confirm that the outcome of any task you have delegated to someone else meets the required standard.

12 Have in place an indemnity arrangement which provides appropriate cover for any practice you take on as a nurse or midwife in the United Kingdom.

To achieve this, you must:

12.1 Make sure that you have an appropriate indemnity arrangement in place relevant to your scope of practice.

Please visit: **www.nmc.org.uk/indemnity.**

Preserve safety

You make sure that patient and public safety is protected. You work within the limits of your competence, exercising your professional 'duty of candour' and raising concerns. Immediately whenever you come across situations that put patients or public safety at risk. You take necessary action to deal with any concerns where appropriate.

13 Recognise and work within the limits of your competence.

To achieve this, you must:

13.1 Accurately assess signs of normal or worsening physical and mental health in the person receiving care.

13.2 Make a timely and appropriate referral to another practitioner when it is in the best interests of the individual needing any action, care or treatment.

13.3 Ask for help from a suitably qualified and experienced healthcare professional to carry out any action or procedure that is beyond the limits of your competence.

13.4 Take account of your own personal safety as well as the safety of people in your care.

13.5 Complete the necessary training before carrying out a new role.

14. Be open and candid with all service users about all aspects of care and treatment, including when any mistakes or harm have taken place.

To achieve this, you must:

14.1 Act immediately to put right the situation if someone has suffered actual harm for any reason or an incident has happened which had the potential for harm.

14.2 Explain fully and promptly what has happened, including the likely effects, and apologise to the person affected and, where appropriate, their advocate, family or care giver.

14.3 Document all these events formally and take further action (escalate) if appropriate so they can be dealt with quickly.

15. Always offer help if an emergency arises in your practice setting or anywhere else.

To achieve this, you must:

15.1 Only act in an emergency within the limits of your knowledge and competence.

15.2 Arrange, wherever possible, for Emergency-Care to be accessed and provided promptly, and.

15.3 Take account of your own safety, the safety of others and the availability of other options for providing care.

16. Act without delay if you believe that there is a risk to patient safety or public protection.

To achieve this, you must:

16.1 Raise and, if necessary, escalate any concerns you may have about patient or public safety, or the level of care people are receiving in your workplace or any other healthcare setting and use the channels available to you in line with our guidance and your local working practices.

16.2 Raise your concerns immediately if you are being asked to practice beyond your role, experience and training.

16.3 Tell someone in authority at the first reasonable opportunity if you experience problems that may prevent you working within the Code or other national standards, taking prompt action to tackle the causes of concern if you can.

16.4 Acknowledge and act on all concerns raised to you, investigating, escalating or dealing with those concerns where it is appropriate for you to do so.

16.5 Not obstruct, intimidate, victimise or in any way hinder a colleague, member of staff, person you care for or member of the public who wants to raise a concern, and

16.6 Protect anyone you have management responsibility for from any harm, detriment, victimisation or unwarranted treatment after a concern is raised.

The professional duty of candour is about openness and honesty when things go wrong. "Every healthcare professional must be open and honest with patients when something goes wrong with their treatment or care which causes, or has the potential to cause, harm or distress." Joint statement from the chief executive of statutory regulators of healthcare professionals.

Please visit: **www.nmc.org.uk/raisingconcerns**

17. Raise concerns immediately if you believe a person is vulnerable or at risk and needs extra support and protection.
To achieve this, you must:
17.1 Take all reasonable steps to protect people who are vulnerable or at risk from harm, neglect or abuse.
17.2 Share information if you believe someone may be at risk of harm, in line with the laws relating to the disclosure of information, and.
17.3 Have knowledge of and keep to the relevant laws and policies about protecting and caring for vulnerable people.

18. Advise on, prescribe, supply, dispense or administer medicines within the limits of your training and competence, the law, our guidance and other relevant policies, guidance and regulations.
To achieve this, you must:
18.1 Prescribe, advice on, or provide medicines or treatment, including repeat prescriptions (only if you are suitably qualified) if you have enough knowledge of that person's health and are satisfied that the medicines or treatment serve that person's health needs.
18.2 Keep to appropriate guidelines when giving advice on using controlled drugs and recording the prescribing, supply, dispensing or administration of controlled drugs.
18.3 Make sure that the care or treatment you advise on, prescribe, supply, dispense or administer for each person is compatible with any other care or treatment they are receiving, including (where possible) over-the-counter medicines.
18.4 Take all steps to keep medicines stored securely, and
18.5 Wherever possible, avoid prescribing for yourself or for anyone with whom you have a close personal relationship.
 Please visit: **www.nmc.org.uk/standards**

19. Be aware of, and reduce as far as possible, any potential for harm associated with your practice.

To achieve this, you must:

19.1 Take measures to reduce as far as possible, the likelihood of mistakes, near misses, harm and the effect of harm if it takes place.

19.2 Take account of current evidence, knowledge and developments in reducing mistakes and the effect of them and the impact of human factors and system failures.

19.3 Keep to and promote recommended practice in relation to controlling and preventing infection, and

19.4 Take all reasonable personal precautions necessary to avoid any potential health risks to colleagues, people receiving care and the public.

Human factors refer to environmental, organisational and job factors, and human and individual characteristics, which influence behaviour at work in a way that can affect health and safety.

Please visit: **www.hse.gov.uk**

Promote professionalism and trust

You uphold the reputation of your profession at all times. You should display a personal commitment to the standards of practice and behaviour set out in the Code. You should be a model of integrity and leadership for others to aspire to. This should lead to trust and confidence in the profession from patients, people receiving care, other healthcare professionals and the public.

20. Uphold the reputation of your profession at all times.

To achieve this, you must:

20.1 Keep to and uphold the standards and values set out in the Code.

20.2 Act with honesty and integrity at all times, treating people fairly and without discrimination, bullying or harassment.

20.3 Be aware at all times of how your behaviour can affect and influence the behaviour of other people.

20.4 Keep to the laws of the country in which you are practicing.

20.5 Treat people in a way that does not take advantage of their vulnerability or cause them upset or distress.

20.6 Stay objective and have clear professional boundaries at all times with people in your care (including those who have been in your care in the past), their families and careers.

20.7 Make sure you do not express your personal beliefs (including political, religious or moral beliefs) to people in an inappropriate way.

20.8 Act as a role model of professional behaviour for students and newly qualified nurses and midwives to aspire.

20.9 Maintain the level of health you need to carry out your professional role, and

20.10 Use all forms of spoken, written and digital communication (including social media and networking sites) responsibly, respecting the right to privacy of others at all times.

Please visit: **www.nmc.org.uk/guidance**

21. Uphold your position as a registered nurse or midwife.

To achieve this, you must:

21.1 Refuse all but the most trivial gifts, favours or hospitality as accepting them could be interpreted as an attempt to gain preferential treatment.

21.2 Never ask for or accept loans from anyone in your care or anyone close to them.

21.3 Act with honesty and integrity in any financial dealings you have with everyone you have a professional relationship with, including people in your care.

21.4 Make sure that any advertisements, publications or published material you produce or have produced for your professional services are accurate, responsible, and ethical, do not mislead or exploit vulnerabilities and accurately reflect your relevant skills, experience and qualifications.

21.5 Never use your professional status to promote causes that are not related to health, and

21.6 Cooperate with the media only when it is appropriate to do so, and then always protecting the confidentiality and dignity of people receiving treatment or care.

22. Fulfil all registration requirements.

To achieve this, you must:

22.1 Meet any reasonable requests so we can oversee the registration process.

22.2 Keep to our prescribed hours of practice and carry out continuing professional development activities, and

22.3 Keep your knowledge and skills up to date, taking part in appropriate and regular learning and professional development activities that aim to maintain and develop your competence and improve your performance.

Please visit: www.nmc.org.uk/standards

23. Cooperate with all investigations and audits.

This includes investigations or audits either against you or relating to others, whether individuals or organisations. It also includes cooperating with requests to act as a witness in any hearing that forms part of an investigation, even after you have left the register.

To achieve this, you must:

23.1 Cooperate with any audit of training records, registration records or other relevant audits that we may want to carry out to make sure you are still fit to practice.

23.2 Tell both us and any employer as soon as you can about any caution or charge against you, or if you have received a conditional discharge in relation to, or have been found guilty of, a criminal offence (other than a protected caution or conviction).

23.3 Tell any employer you work for if you have had your practice restricted or had any other conditions imposed on you by us or any other relevant body.

23.4 Tell us and your employers at the first reasonable opportunity if you are or have been disciplined by any regulatory or licensing organisation, including those who operate outside of the professional healthcare environment, and

23.5 Give your NMC Pin when any reasonable request for it is made.

Please visit: **www.nmc.org.uk**

24. Respond to any complaints made against you professionally.
To achieve this, you must:
24.1 Never allow someone's complaint to affect the care that is provided to them, and
24.2 Use all complaints as a form of feedback and an opportunity for reflection and learning to improve practice.

25. Provide leadership to make sure people's wellbeing is protected and to improve their experiences of the healthcare system.
To achieve this, you must:
25.1 Identify priorities, manage time, staff and resources effectively and deal with risk to make sure that the quality of care or service you deliver is maintained and improved, putting the needs of those receiving care or services first, and
25.2 Support any staff you may be responsible for to follow the Code at all times. They must have the knowledge, skills and competence for safe practice; and understand how to raise any concerns linked to any circumstances where the Code has, or could be, broken.
When telling your employers, this includes telling (i) any person, body or organisation you are employed by, or intend to be employed by, as a nurse or midwife; and (ii) any person, body or organisation with whom you have an arrangement to provide services as a nurse or midwife.

Obligations of health care professionals
The obligation of an employer, manager and healthcare professional is to:
- Ensure that what is actually done is done safely and appropriately.
- Make clear what cannot be done, or at least be done safely.
- Ensure the patient is treated with the appropriate urgency.

What is the NMC Code?
- The NMC has updated its Code of professional standards.
- The revised Code became effective on 31 March 2015 and all registered nurses and midwives are required to uphold its standards of practice and behaviours.
- The Code is centred on four themes, with public protection at the core, and builds on the existing foundation of good nursing and midwifery practice.
- The Code should be used as a 'living' guide at the heart of everyday nursing and midwifery practice.

NMC Standard of Conduct

NMC (2008) the Code: Standard of Conduct, Performance and Ethics for Nurses and Midwives
- As a professional, you are personally accountable for your actions and omissions in your practice and must always be able to justify your decisions.
- You must always act lawfully, whether those laws relate to your professional practice or personal life.
- Failure to comply with this Code may bring your fitness to practice into question and endanger your registration.

Nursing Theorists

When assessing, planning, implementing & evaluating the care that we give, we need to ensure that it is evidence based and that it will benefit our patients.

1. Virginia Henderson – Need Theory.
2. Martha Rogers – Unitary Human Beings.
3. Dorothy E. Orem – Self-care Theory.
4. Betty Neuman – The System Model.
5. Hildegard Peplau – Interpersonal Theory.
6. Madeleine Leininger – Transcultural Nursing.
7. Patricia Benner – From Novice to Expert.

In **Contingency Theory** - the way you manage care should change accordance to the circumstances and conditions of the patients. One size doesn't fit all.

Nutritional Status

What are methods used in assessing Nutritional Status?
 a. Body weight and weight loss. Body mass Index (BMI)
 b. Skinfold thickness.
 c. Dietary intake and biochemical investigations.
 d. Chemical exoneration.

If a client has a total parenteral nutrition (TPN) infused at 40mL per hour. The nurse then ran out of fluid prior to a new bag expected at the clinic. What would be the most Important, for the nurse to assess at the time with the client?
If the bag runs dry and another concentration of dextrose is hung, the nurse should assess for hypoglycemia which is the major concern.

O

Observation

What is Observation?

Observation is the conscious deliberate use of the physical senses to gather data from the patient and their environment.

Physical Assessment /Examination

Is the systematic assessment of all body systems and is concerned with identifying strengths weakness and defects in a patient's functional ability.

Osmotic Pressure

What is Osmotic Pressure?

The amount of solute in a solution determined the osmolality. In other words, the higher the solute concentration, the higher the osmolality known as **Osmotic Pressure.**

The movement of water and solutes out of intravascular space and into the interstitial space is dependent on opposing factor: **osmotic and hydrostatic pressure.**

The **O.P** is provided by plasma protein that is too large to pass through the membrane even under pressure.

Oedema can result if the membrane becomes permeable to protein. When **O.P** is reduced, it results in excess of water moving into the **interstitial space.**

Oxygen Therapy

What are the indications of Oxygen Therapy?

1. COPD.
2. Pulmonary fibrosis.
3. Heart failure.
4. Severe long term Asthma.
5. Pulmonary hypertension.
6. Cystic fibrosis.
7. Obesity related to hypo ventilation.

What are the precautions to take before or while administering Oxygen?
1. There should be no smoking.
2. Keep oxygen six feet or more from heat sources e.g. Gas cooker.
3. Do not use flammable liquids e.g. aerosols, paint thinner, cleaning fluid.
4. Do not use Vaseline or oil based emollient.
5. Make sure you have installed smoke detectors and fire alarm.
6. Inform the fire fighters that you have oxygen at home.
7. Always keep oxygen cylinders upright.

What is Home Oxygen Therapy?
Home Oxygen Therapy involves breathing in air that contains more oxygen than normal from a cylinder or machine in your home.
This is prescribed if your lungs or heart does not receive inadequate supply due to a condition. Oxygen is administered through:
1. Nasal canals.
2. Pocket mask with oxygen port.
3. Self-inflating resuscitation bag with oxygen reservoir.
4. Ambubag mask.
5. Mask with one way value.

P

Patient Safety

What is Patient Safety?

It is the number one priority and implies the prevention of harm to patients.

- The freedom from accidental or preventable injuries produced by medical or nursing care.
- A system of care delivery that prevents errors and an ability to learn from the errors that occurred.

  S ---- Sense of error.

  A ---- Acts to prevent.

  F ---- Follow safety guidelines.

  E ---- Enquires into accidents and death.

  T ---- Take appropriate action.

  Y---- Your responsibility.

Safety of What?

1. Safety of Place involves; Infrastructure, Fire, Electrical, and Mechanical.
2. Safety of Property involves; Equipment, Material and storage.
3. Safety of People involves; Patients, Staff and Visitors.

What are the Safety Goals?

1. Identify your patient correctly.
2. Improve an effective communication channel.
3. Improve the safety of High-alert Medications.
4. Eliminate wrong procedure for surgeries.
5. Reduce the risk of acquired infections.
6. Reduce the risk of patients' harm resulting from fall.

Note: Please do not harm any patient irrespective of the race, gender, culture, beliefs, colour and language etc. Safety is everyone's responsibility.

Peak Flow Test

What is Peak Flow Test?

Peak Flow is a simple measurement of how quickly you can blow air out of the lungs. Usually it is used for accessing and monitoring asthma.

Actually measuring the rate and how quickly or fast one is able to breath out. The peak flow scores indicate if airways are narrowed which a sign of asthma is.

The scores show if the condition is improving or worsening in asthma attack. Peak Flow detects if a particular event triggers the symptoms.

How do you measure Peak Flow?

A. Sit or stand in a comfortable position.
B. Set the meter to "0".
C. The meter should be held horizontally and do not obstruct the measurement scale.
D. Place your lips tightly around the mouth piece and breath in deep air.
E. Breathe out quickly.
F. Take note of your reading.
G. Repeat three times.
H. The highest of the three measurements should be recorded as the score, read as (1/min) liters/minute.

What is another name for Peak Flow?

Peak Expiratory Flow.

Peripheral Venous Device

This is a device used to draw blood or give treatments, nutritional supplements or fluids. This is usually done with a catheter as the device.

What are the guidelines for the Peripheral Venous Device?

A Gastrostomy (G- tube) is inserted in the stomach to deliver nutritional supplements.

Targets are:
- To identify the type of therapy suitable administered.
- Duration of therapy.
- Catheter gauge or size.
- Vascular assessment.
- Patient's preference and value.

Site Selections are:
- Cephalic.
- Accessory of cephalic.
- Upper cephalic.
- Median antebrachial..
- Median cubital.
- Ante cubital.
- Ante cubital fossa.

Preliminary/ Initial Stage in the procedure requires you to:
- Assess the environment.
- Gather equipment.
- Hand hygiene.
- Choose the insertion site.
- Prepare the site.

Peripheral Maintenance

Peripheral Maintenance is assessed and based on:
- Catheter patency.
- Catheter stabilization.
- Catheter dressing.
- Catheter anchoring.
- Assessment, monitoring and removal.
- Documentation.

Midline Catheters used are:
- **3- 8** inches long.
- Single or dual lumen.
- Placed in the basalic, cephalic or median cubital veins.
- Ideal if duration of therapy is expected for 1-4 weeks.
- Inserted via sterile techniques by experienced nurses.

Pharmacology Targets

What is Pharmacology?

Pharmacology is a branch of science that deals with the interaction of drugs within the living organisms or the study of pharmacokinetics and pharmacodynamics.

What is a Drug?

A drug is any chemical entity that causes a change in biological function in living organisms. Some drugs are formed inside the body such as insulin and noradrenalin etc. Drugs that are introduced into the body from outside are called Xenobiotic.

What is a Dose?

A specific amount of drug prescribed to be at one time.

What is Blood Brain Barrier?

It is a tight endothelial cells of the brain capillaries and cells of the brain around the capillaries that doesn't allow the passage of certain lipid insoluble substances to pass from the blood into the brain. Liquid drugs can easily cross this barrier. Examples of lipid soluble drugs are: Diazepam, Thiopental, and Phenobarbital.

What is Volume of Distribution?

The total volume of the body fluid in which a drug appears to be distributed according to its concentration in the blood or plasma .VD of a drug can be determined by the following formula.

V. D. (Volume of Distribution).

=Total Amount of drug in the body /concentration of the blood plasma.

What is Potency?

It is the weight of the drug that produces a certain magnitude of response. For example; the lesser the weight of blood require to produce a given effect, the more its potency. E.g. Clonidine produces its antihypertensive effect in 0.2 – 0.3mg daily dose. While antihypertensive dose of Methyldopa is 500 – 2000mg per day. Thus Clonidine is more potent than Methyldopa.

What is Efficacy?

If the dose of a drug is increased its effect will be increased proportionately, until a stage is reached. Beyond that there is no further increase in effect that will occur, even if a large dose of that drug is given. The maximum of the drug beyond which further increase in its effect occurs, even if the dose of that drug is increased to a large amount is called efficacy. Example: Morphine is more effective in severe types of pain while Aspirin is effective in mild to moderate pain.

What is Therapeutic Index?

The ratio between median toxic dose (TD50) and median effective dose (ED50) is called therapeutic index. Therapeutic index = TD50/ED50.

What is Idiosyncrasy?

It is a rare type of response to a drug that is not related to its dose, that, even a small dose of it can cause that response. For example, a rare adverse effect with Chloramphenicol is aplastic anaemia.

What is Hypersensitivity?

Allergic or immunological response to a drug. For example anaphylactic shock with penicillin is a severe type of hypersensitivity reaction.

What is Tolerance?

Repeated use of a drug that causes gradual decrease to the response of that drug. E.g. Chronic use of Morphine will decrease many of its effect in the body; therefore the dose of the drug has to be increased as the time progresses to maintain the usual effects of that drug.

What is a Receptor?

Receptors are macromolecules (big molecules). Most of the receptors are protein in nature. They are mostly those drugs that act on the cells which bind to the receptors. Those which bind to the receptors and show their effect are called organists, while some drugs binds to the receptors but don't produce any effect. These drugs are known as an antagonist as they prevent the binding of agonists with the receptors.

What is the Adverse Drug Reaction?

Drugs may produce two types of effects i.e. adverse drug reaction or undesired effect. This effect may range from the mild type of adverse effect to server effect that may cause the death of the person. Adverse drug reaction may be classified into the following types;

- Idiosyncrasy.
- Drug allergy.
- Direct toxic effect.
- Drug dependence.
- Tolerance.

What is Shock?

It is a clinical condition in which there is an inadequate supply of blood to the tissues. It causes hypotension, oliguria, and metabolic acidosis. The following are the common types of shock:

a. Hypovolemic shock
b. Septic shock.
c. Cardiogenic shock.
d. Anaphylactic shock.

What is Drug Clearance?

It can be defined as the volume of blood or plasma required to clear the drug in a unit or period of time. Thus, to determine clearance we have to find that volume of blood or plasma from which drug is removed during a unit or period of time. By removal of drug, we mean the metabolism and excretion of drug. If we know the clearance of the drug we can adjust its dose properly. Clearance of the drug can be determined by the following formula:

CI = Rate of elimination   where CI is clearance.
Concentration of drug in the blood

What is Drug Excretion?
Removal of drugs from the body is known as their excretion. Drugs are excreted from the body either in the form of their metabolites or in exchanged form. Excretion can occur from the following routes;
   a) Faecal.
   b) Renal.
   c) Biliary.
   d) Pulmonary.
Others are: sweat, saliva, breastmilk etc.

What is Toxicology?
It is an aspect of pharmacology that deals with the adverse effect of drugs on living organisms. In addition to drugs used in the therapy, it also deals with many other chemicals that may be responsible for the household, environmental, or industrial intoxication.

What is an Antidote?
An antidote is any substance which is used to oppose the effects of poisons without causing any damage to the body. For example, antidote for Benzodiazepine is Flumazenil.

What is Bioavailability?
It can be define as a fraction of unmodified drug reaching into the systemic circulation after it is administered by any route. IV administration of drugs produces 100% bioavailability as a whole of the drug enters the systemic circulation. Oral administration of the drug may not produce 100% bioavailability due to incomplete absorption of a drug from the gastrointestinal tract and due to first pass effect of some of the drugs.

Fentanyl drugs are Opioids. It is 100 times stronger than Morphine. Indications for Fentanyl Drugs include:

- Anxiety reduction.
- General mood lift.
- Sedation.
- Pain relief.
- Euphoria.
- Relaxation

It is used for acute chronic pain.

Side effects:
- Drowsiness.
- Vomiting.
- Nausea.
- Constipation.
- Sweating.
- Decreased blood pressure.
- Respiratory depression.
- Difficulty in urinating.

Short acting anesthesia, breakthrough pain transdermal use for extended pain relief, cardiovascular stability intravenous -30-60 minutes, and onset from the second minutes.

Transdermal: 72-hours (total), onset -1 to 4 hours.

Intranasal: 1-3 hours, onset 5 – 10 minutes.

Buccal: 1 -3 hours, onset10 – 15 minutes.

Premenopausal Syndrome

In the average, women enter menopause as from the age of 50 years. But transition into menopause is a gradual process before that stage; they experience certain symptoms known as Premenopausal Syndrome. During this transition, the ovaries begin to produce fewer estrogens. It starts in a woman in her 40's but can be earlier in some women. The average length of premenopausal is 4 years.

The Premenopausal Syndrome includes:

- Irregular menses.
- Hot flushes and night sweats.
- Loss of sex drive.
- Breast tenderness.
- Fatigue.
- Vaginal dryness.
- Mood swings.
- Urinary urgency.
- Sleeplessness.
- Headaches.
- Nausea.
- Weight gain.
- Dizziness.
- Anxiety.

Most women experience the symptoms a year after menopause.
Women can still get pregnant during their premenopausal syndrome.

Premenopausal syndrome should not cause fear, since it's not a disease. It is a normal part of a women's natural life cycle which simply indicates transition to menopause.

Pre-operative Care

What is Pre-operative Care?

Pre-operative care refers to a nursing care provided to a patient before a surgical operation commence.

What are the required steps for a nurse to take in the Pre-operative Care?

- Assess physical, psychological and social statutes of the patient.
- Prepare patient for surgery.
- Implement nursing Interventions.
- Pre-operative history and physical assessment may be done at the doctor's office, hospital pre-admission area, Inpatient unit of the hospital, outpatient, and the main surgery unit or on the phone.
- Identify Individual's at risk for post or Intra operations complications in other to implement Interventions.

What is the Pre-operative Checklist?

- Patient ID confirmed
- ID band
- Allergies
- Procedure & site verifications
- Consent signed
- Jewelry removed
- Valuables secured.
- Advance directives required or not.

Pressure Ulcer

What is Pressure Ulcer?

Pressure Ulcers are injuries or a break in the continuity of the skin and underlying tissues, caused by prolonged pressure on the skin. It usually affects people or patient confined to the bed or chair for a long period of time.

What are the symptoms of pressure ulcers?

a. Pain in the affected area.
b. 1st stage – A patch skin that feels warmth, and does not Blanche
c. 2nd stage of pressure ulcer - Is an open wound or blisters. It causes damage to the epidermis or dermis.
d. 3rd stage pressure ulcer- A deep wound that reaches the deeper layers of the skin.
e. 4th stage pressure ulcer- A very deep wound that reaches the muscles, tissues and ligaments.

What are the treatments of Pressure Ulcer?

1. Change position 2 hourly.
2. Eat healthy food, mostly fruits and vegetables rich in vitamin C. and protein rich food.
3. A special mattress or foam.
4. Debridement.

Prions

What are Prions?

Prions are infectious agents that consist entirely of protein aggregates. These agents are responsible for Mad Cow disease in cattle, Scrapie in sheep and Creutzfeldt–Jakob (CJD) disease in human.

In the case of CJD, the proteins end up killing off many nerve cells, which eventually degenerates brain function. Patients with these conditions develop a sponge –resembling brain which is a cluster of dead neurons. Human prions diseases are usually transmissible, but not efficiently shed and taken up by others to initiate new infections.

What are the Symptoms?
1. Insomnia.
2. Impaired judgments.
3. Visual disturbances.
4. Depression.
5. Memory disorders.
6. Thinking.
7. Undergo personality changes.

What are the causes of Prions?
The gene in the DNA encodes the prions protein causing the abnormal brain damage, prions with its mutation in the gene passes through the egg to the offspring.

The diagnoses are:
- MRI.
- CT scan.
- Spinal fluid test to rule out meningitis.

How can Prions be transmitted?
It is by coming in contact with infected brain tissues, spinal fluid and infected blood and blood products. Standard precautions should be practiced.

Professional Boundary
What is Boundary?
A boundary is a limit you can set on what you will accept of another person's words or action.
Boundaries can be:
- Material
- Physical
- Mental
- Emotional

Healthy boundaries and respect help people communicate more effectively and work together, making people less likely to leave their relationships. So take care of yourself before taking care of others.

What is Professional Boundaries?
It is a limit to which the nurse-patient relationship should be without crossing the bridge of neither trust nor take advantage of the situation presented to you professionally.

It also means;
Boundary crossing that is: -
- Inadvertent
- Purposeful.
- Perceived need.

Boundary crossing or Boundary drift leads to Boundary violations.

What does Professional Boundary Violations means?
- Excessive personal disclosure.
- Secrecy.
- Reversal of roles.
- Sexual misconduct which is a part of boundary violation that involves:
  i. Seduction.
  ii. Sexually demeaning.
  iii. Harassing.

Are interpreted as sexual misconduct to the patient. This leads to a bridge of trust.

How can you recognize warning signs of boundary violations?
They are:
- Excessive self – disclosure.
- Secretive behaviour.
- Special treatment.
- Flirtation.
- Over protective behaviour.

Many of these behaviours may indicate having a shift from therapeutic nurse – patient relationship to over involvement.

How should nurses treat their patients?
Nurses are expected to treat their patients:
- Professionally.
- Objectively and.
- Actively.

What is the implication to Nursing Practice?
Boundary crossing can happen to any nurse. Nurses who put their needs ahead of their patients' needs will cross over these boundaries. This is a serious violation in nursing practice.

Protective Foods
What is a Protective Food?
Protective foods are foods rich in Vitamins and Minerals. It protects us from diseases and infections.
Green vegetables such as Spinach, Carrot and fruits have lots of vitamins and minerals.

Pulmonary Embolism
What are the signs of Pulmonary Embolism?
1. Trouble catching your breath or breathing fast for no reason.
2. Pain in the chest which may worsen when taking a deep breath.
3. A fast heart rate for no reason (palpitation).
4. Dizziness faints or pass out.
5. Haemoptysis.

Purulent
The term "Purulent" is often used in regard to drainage (pus and mucus).

R
Record Keeping
What is Good Record Keeping?

The Code of Professional Conduct (NMC, 2002a) advises that good note keeping is the vital tool of communication between nurses and must; ensure that the care record for the patient or client is an accurate account of treatment, care planning and delivery.

Importance of Record Keeping

Record keeping whether electronic, audio or visual is used to monitor a client progress and communicate with other care providers. It also reflects the nursing care that is provided to a client; prioritize on these rounds; medication and treatments.

Round includes introduction, assessment, vital signs, pain assessment, special request, and concern. Do not hesitate to stop and document after each contact.

Medication – all medications; food and drinks, bath room trips. Tell your patient what you are given them, this develops trust, attend to other requests. Keep record and document.

Treatment contacts- It includes, ambulation, incentive spirometer, wound care, attendance to more request and document.

Respiratory Disorder
Mention the types of Respiratory Disorder?
- Flu cold.
- Asthma.
- Emphysema.
- Chronic Bronchitis.

Respiratory Failure
What are the indications for Respiratory Failure?
They are:
- Coma.
- Severe.
- Injury.
- Paralysis.
- Pneumonia, Cystic fibrosis (This conditions damages the lungs), Neuron diseases or Guillain-Barre's Syndrome.

Revalidation
What Is Revalidation?
Revalidation is a process of showing you are living and abiding by the Codes and standard of practice and behaviour. It builds on the previous preparatory requirements. This process is observed every three years at the point of renewal of registration in UK.

Benefits of Revalidation
To the NMC:
- It helps to strengthen the regulation of nurses and midwives.
- It helps to raise standard of practice.
- Provide more insight into how nursing and midwifery professionals are practiced.

To the Employers:
- Increases confidence that their staff practice safely and effectively.
- Encourage more consistent participation in appraisal and professional development.

For Nurses and Midwives:
- Raise awareness of the Code and standards that are expected of nurses and midwives.
- Encourage a culture of sharing, reflection and continuous improvement.
- Encourage nurses to stay up to date in their professional practice.

For the Public:
- Provide confidence that nurses and midwives are up to date in terms of their skills and professional development.
- Provide assurance that nurses and midwives are being regularly reviewed.

Risk Assessment

Risk is an uncertain future event or the mission objective; it could have a positive or negative effect. Risk is the chance of damage or harm occurring.

A hazard is a source of potential damage or harm.

Likelihood is the chance of an events occurring.

Consequence is the most likely outcome.

Control measures are actions that can be taken to reduce a risk.

Residual risk is the risk remaining after control measures are in place.

Define Risk Assessment?

Risk assessment is a careful examination of what could cause harm to people in the workplace.

What are the steps to a Risk Assessment?
1. Looking for hazards.
2. Deciding who might be harmed and how.
3. Evaluating the risk and deciding whether the existing precautions are adequate or whether more should be done.
4. Record your findings and tell your employees about them.
5. Review your assessment if it is necessary, For example, if there is an accident, or if work changes significantly or injury occurs or when someone returns to work after sickness or probably suffer a change in their health that could affect or be affected by their work.

Why do you need Risk assessment?
1. Risk assessment form an integral part of a good occupational health and safety management plan.
2. They help to create awareness of hazard and risks.
3. Identify who may be at risk (patient, nurse, doctor, visitor's, cleaners, lab technicians, maintenance, children, pharmacists and radiologists. etc.)
4. They determine if existing control measure are adequate or if more should be done.
5. They prevent injuries or illness when done at the design or planning stage.
6. They prioritize hazards and control measure.
7. To be sure that all hazards are found.
8. It Includes: an assessment of groups that may have a different level of risk such as inexperience workers, persons with disability or expectant mothers, and the elderly ones.
9. Look out for unusual conditions that may be unavailable, an employee's situation, e.g. power outage etc.
10. It is important to carry out a risk assessment because if someone gets hurt, the organization or institution may likely be sued in the court for damages.

S

Safeguarding Vulnerable Adult
What is Safeguarding Vulnerable Adult?
We are so responsible for caring for those who are not able to care for themselves, to share information or concern.

The 4 "R"s of Safeguarding
- Recognise.
- Respond.
- Report.
- Record.

Safeguarding adults involve; "protecting an adult's right to live in safety, free from abuse and neglect. It includes ensuring: quality of life, dignity, gives respect and respects their choices.

What can you do to stay safe in the hospital?
Preventable infections, mix-ups and other errors are ways or factors affecting safety measure.
Talk to your doctor on how you can stay safe in a particular facility.

a. Bring a family member or friend to check in and or discharge from the hospital.
b. Be alert and say something, keep track of what is happening. Ask questions such as "Did you wash your hand"?
c. Know your medications and the prescriptions, adverse effect as well as reasons for administering it.
d. Ensure names and other details are correct.

Self-Harm
What is Self-Harm?
It is when somebody intentionally inflict pains to his/her body. It is usually a way of coping with or expressing overwhelming emotional distress.

Sepsis
What is Sepsis?
Sepsis is a serious condition in which the body's reaction to an infection damages the organs and tissues.

What are the treatments for Sepsis?
  a. Antibiotics.
  b. Intravenous fluids.
  c. Oxygen.
  d. Intake and output.
  e. Vital signs
  f. Blood cultures.

Septic Shock
What is Septic Shock?
It occurs when the blood pressure drops to a dangerous level (hypotension) as a result of the dilatation of the blood vessels after an infection. This is a threatening condition, the body response slow down. Hence, the amount of blood in circulation is reduced, stopping the body's organ from working properly.
Sepsis is a serious condition that happens when the body's reaction to an infection damages its own organs.
What are the symptoms of Septic Shock?
Light-headedness (dizziness)
  • Confusion.
  • Feeling sick and vomiting.
  • Shortness of breath.
  • Muscular pain.
  • Sluggish speech.
  • Oliguria.
  • Cold, clammy and pace or mottled skin.
  • Loss of consciousness.

Mention or list major treatments for Septic Shock.
  a. Fluids for rehydration
  b. Antibiotics against infections, bactericidal
  c. Oxygen to boost the level of oxygen level in the blood
  d. Ventilator. For airway patency.
  e. Surgery to remove the source of the infection (abscess).
  f. Administration of medicines that increase blood pressure and help blood to reach the tissues and organs.

What are the indications for Septic Shock?
It is more common to:
- Babies.
- Elderly people.
- Pregnant women.
- Diabetes.
- Liver cirrhosis.
- Kidney disease.
- Cancer.
- HIV or AIDS.
- Chemotherapy patients.
- Long time steroids treatment.
- People with low immunity.
- Extreme loss of blood.

Serous Fluid or Serosal Fluid
Where can Serous Fluid are found?
The term "Serous Fluid" or "Serosal Fluid" is used for various body fluids that are typically pale, yellow and transparent, which fills inside the body cavities.

Serous-Sanguineous
What is the meaning of Serous-sanguineous?
Serous-sanguineous means containing or relating to blood components and the liquid part of blood (serum). Whereas Sanguineous contain only blood.

Shock
What is Shock?
Shock or Hypo-perfusion is the inability of the circulatory system to supply cells with oxygen.

What are the signs of Compensated Shock?
- Increased heart rate.
- Increased respiration.
- Constriction of peripheral circulation.
- Pale, cool skin.

What are the signs of Decompensated Shock?
- Low blood volume.
- Lack of perfusion.
- Reduced blood pressure.

What are the signs of Irreversible Shock?
- Perfusion to Organs cannot be restored.
- Cells damage.
- Irreparably damaged Organs.

List 3 major types of Shock?
- Cardiogenic shock.
- Hypovolemic shock.
- Neurogenic shock.

Sickle Cell Disease
What are the symptoms of Sickle Cell Disease?
- Pain.
- Infection.
- Tiredness, shortness of breath.
- Some people develop strokes.
- Anaemia.

Mention the causes of SCD

Faulty genes inherited from parents, it affects mostly Africans, Asians, and the Middle Eastern populations.

Source Isolation
What is Source of Isolation?

Source isolation is the term used to describe the physical isolation of patients with infections, to reduce or prevent the spread of micro-organism from an infected/colonized patient to susceptible individual. It indicates that the patient is the "source of isolation". (Wilson 2003).

Spinal Cord Size

What is the size of Spinal Cord?

The spinal cord is about 45cm in length and extends from the base of the brain to the caudal vertebrae.

Subjective Data

How do you determine a Subjective data?

Subjective data includes the client's, sensations, feelings, and perception of health status. Subjective data can only be affected by the person.

Suicide

What are the warning signs of Suicide?

Suicide is the act of working towards ending one's life.

Successful warnings are:

- Talk or write about death, dying or suicide.
- Actually, looking for means to kill themselves, such as keeping many tablets to swallow.
- Self-isolate

What are the preventions of Suicide?

Exercise, Diet; Music, Social activities

- It helps to lift your mood.
- Reduce stress and anxiety.
- Improved self-esteem.
- Encourage the release of feed – good chemical called endorphins.
- Don't drink more than the recommended daily limit of alcohol, 3% a day, for women.
- Drug misuse or abuse can increase your risk of developing a serious mental health.
- Avoid isolation.
- Staying positive.
- Self-help.

Supervision

What is Supervision?

Nursing supervision is the delegation, by monitoring the performance of the risk or function and assures compliance with standard of practice, policies and procedure. Level and nature of monitoring vary with needs of clients and experience of the assistant.

T

Thyroiditis

What is Thyroiditis?

It is the inflammation of the thyroid gland, which causes high or low levels of thyroid hormones in the blood. Thyroid hormones affect heart rate and body temperature.

What are the types of Thyroiditis?

   I.   **Hashimoto's Thyroiditis.**
- a. Caused by immune system attacking the thyroid gland making it to be inflamed and damaged. Over time the thyroid is destroyed leading to hypo thyroiditis. This causes the symptoms of underactive thyroid gland.
- b. Weight again, dry skin tiredness.
- c. The inflamed thyroid causes goiter.

   II.   **De quervain's (sub-acute) Thyroiditis.**
- a. Tender and painful neck, jaw or ear.
- b. Leads to hyperthyroid causing anxiety, insomnia and heat palpitation.

   III.   **Postpartum Thyroiditis.**

Common in women with type 2 diabetes, a few women who has given birth, manifest symptoms of hyperthyroidism few weeks later, leading to hypothyroidism.

   IV.   **Painless Thyroiditis.**

It affects both women and men.

V. **Drug induced Thyroiditis.**
Certain drugs damage the thyroid gland.
VI. **Radiated - induced Thyroiditis.**
VII. **Acute infections Thyroiditis.**

Hypothyroidism - Does not produce enough hormones due to the auto immune system attacking the thyroid gland and damages it.
Hyperthyroidism - Product of excessive thyroid hormones occurs mostly in women between the ages of 20- 40 years.

What are the Symptoms of Thyroiditis?
- Nervousness, anxiety and irritability.
- Mood swings.
- Persistent tiredness weakness.
- Sensitivity to heat.
- Enlarged thyroid gland.
- Palpitations.
- Twitching.
- Weight loss.

Causes of thyroiditis: Graves' diseases, some medications, lump. If not treated well, it can lead to bulging of the eyes, pre-ecchymosis, a life threatening condition.

Tracheostomy
Why is Tracheostomy used?
A tracheotomy is needed if unable to breathe normally due to underlying health condition or due to blocked airway.
It delivers oxygen to the lungs when the patient can't breathe normally (Respiratory Failure).

What are the indications for Tracheostomy?
They are:
- Blockages - using tracheostomy to bypass an air way.
- Breathing problem - a tracheostomy can deliver oxygen to the patient's lung if he can't breathe normally.

- Removing fluid - tracheostomy is carried out to remove fluid that built up in the airways, unable to cough out well, lung infection, Pneumonia,
- Muscular weakness or paralysis.
- Air ways filled with blood as a result of injury.

U

Unconditional Positive Regard
What is meant by the term "Unconditional Positive Regard"?
According to humanistic "Psychologist Carl Rogers", it is the basic acceptance and support of a person, regardless of what the person says or does.
Accepting and supporting a person, regardless of what they have said or done.
Accepting a person, regardless of what the person said or does.

Unconsciousness
Unconsciousness- is a physiological state in which the patient is unresponsive to sensory stimuli and lack awareness of self and the environment (Hickey 2000).

Urinary Incontinence
Define Urinary Incontinence
It is an unintentional passing of urine.

What are the causes of the various types of Urinary Incontinence?
  a. **Stress Incontinence** is caused as a result of weak pelvic floor muscles and the urethral sphincter.
  b. **Urge Incontinence** is caused as a result of over activity of the detrusor muscle, which control the bladders.
  c. **Overflow Incontinence** is caused as a result of obstruction to the bladders.
  d. **Congenital or Total Incontinence** is caused as a result of bladder fistula from birth, spinal injury.

What are the risk factors for Urinary Incontinence?
- Age.
- Neurological condition e.g. spinal cord injury.
- Surgical procedures (hysterectomy, pelvic surgery).
- Diabetes.
- Physical trauma.
- Menopause.
- Cystitis and UTI.
- Enlargement of the prostrate (benign prostatic hyperplasia).
- Prostrate surgery.
- Prostate cancer.

V

Validation
What is Validation?
It is the process of confirming that data are actual and factual.

Venous Thrombosis
What are the causes of Venous Thrombosis?
1. Not moving about for a long time, such as a long trip. Sitting in a particular position longer than 2 hours at a stretch.
2. Staying in bed because of sickness or as a result of generalized body weakness or Injury.
3. Staying in the hospital or having surgery such as hip or knee surgery.
4. Other risk factors are: overweight, smoking, Injury or trauma.
5. Blood clots
6. Cancer.
7. Birth control.
8. Childbirth.
9. Old age.
10. Birth control pills.

Diagnosing of Venous Thrombosis blood clots using:
1. Ultrasound.
2. Blood test for d-dimer.
3. CT scan.
4. Ventilation – perfusion lung (VQ) scan.

What signs are manifested in Venous Thromboembolism?
- Swelling (usually in one leg or arm).
- Skin that is red or not showing the usual colour/complexion.
- Warmth in the area that is swollen.

Vulnerable Adults
Who are Vulnerable Adults?
Some older adults are more vulnerable than others due to:-
- Isolation.
- Illness.
- Memory problem.
- Turbulent relationships.
- Age.
- Disability.
- Mental Health/ Mental capacity.
- Difficulty in handling self-care.

Recognise various forms of abuse and be aware of the warning signs of abuse.

Answer these questions,
Which form of abuse is most commonly experienced by vulnerable adults?
Neglect or physical abuse.
Answer: Neglect.

W

Walker Techniques with Injured Leg

How can a patient use a walker with the injured leg?

1. Step forward with your injured leg
2. Use the walker to help keep your balance.
3. Bring the other foot forward to the centre of the walker.
4. Move the walker forward to start the next step.

Which nursing assessment is the most important regarding proper fitting of crutches?

The crutches should be positioned about 2 inches under the axillary area to prevent nerve damage to the brachial plexus area which would may result in the paralysis of the arm.

After the amputation of the left above-the-knee, what response by the client regarding positioning that indicates the clients understand the importance of prone position postoperatively?

The response should be, " I need to lie on my stomach it will help me from getting a flexion contracture at my left hip". The prone position provides maximum extension of the hip joint and prevents hip flexion contracture. If the hip contracture occurs, it might be very difficult to correctly it in prosthesis.

Waste Colour

What are the Waste Colour codes?

They are:

1. Yellow – Waste that requires disposal by incineration.
2. Orange – Waste which may be treated.
3. Purple – Cytotoxic and Cytostatic waste.
4. Yellow / Black – Offensive / Hygienic waste.
5. Red – Anatomical waste for incineration.
6. Black – Domestic (municipal waste).
7. Blue – Medical waste for incineration.
8. White – Amalgam waste for recovery.

Wound Healing
What are the stages of Wound Healing?
Stages of Wound Healing

Stage1 wound - Do not have any visible skin cuts. However, the skin covering the wound can be remarkably different from the surrounding area.

Stage 2 wound - The topmost layers of skin is damaged (epidermis and dermis). There may be some drainage.

Stage 3 wound- Wounds are deeper than stage 2 wounds. It typically damages the "fatty" layer (subcutaneous) and muscles but do not extend any further. There may be dead tissue and drainage.

Stages 4wound - Wounds are characterized by deeper damage down to the bone, blood vessels, nerves and muscles. Dead tissue and drainage are almost always present.

Wound Management

What is a Wound?
A wound is a disruption of the normal structure and function of the skin.

What are the principles of Wound Management?
  a. **Types of Wound**
- Abrasion.
- Puncture.
- Laceration.
- Incision.

  b. **Assessment ; History**
- Mechanism.
- Site.
- Time.
- Place.
- Allergies,
- Current medication,
- Tetanus Immunization.
- Implants (E.g. Arthroplasties).
- Occupation/ hobbies.

Examination
- Wound measurements: length, width, death of wound.
- Wound bed – tissue type visible (e.g. necrotic gelation).
- Evidence of contamination, non- visible tissue of foreign bodies.
- Condition of the surrounding skin.
- Signs of infection.
- Involvement of deep structure (e.g. muscle, nerve).
- Type and amount of exude, if present.
- Odour if present.
- Swab.

Feel
- Test sensation.
- Current pain status.

Move
- Test muscles and tendon functions whilst observing the wound.

Wound Cleaning and Closure

- Primary closure – immediately, neatest scar, risk for infection.
- Delayed primary closure – 48 hours delay with the antibiotics.
- Secondary healing – allow wound to heal itself slowly, increased risk of infection.

Wound Closure

- Suture –non absorbable.
- Tissue glue.
- Adhesive strips.
- Skin staple.
- Dressing
- Avoid excessive tension.
- Removal time- scarring verses strengthening.
- Generally – 7 days.
- Facially – 4- 5 days.
- Lower limbs and exterior surfaces of joints – up to 14 days.

Indications for Tetanus

- 6 hours old at presentation.
- Depth and length (e.g. puncture / stab wounds).
- Containing devitalized tissue.
- Possible contaminated with soil or manure.
- Showing clinical evidence of sepsis.
- Give tetanus toxoid vaccine.

What are the Interventions of highest priority to give to a patient who arrives at the emergency department with a penetrating chest wound and a rush of air through the trauma site?

In a chronological order these are the step.

a. Place air-occlusive dressing over the chest wound to prevent further complications such as pneumothorax, Mediastinal shift.
b. Administer oxygen and begin to set up the tube insertions.
c. Monitor blood gases to determine early acid-base imbalance.
d. Medicate for pain with caution so as not to depress the respiratory center.

Y

Yellow Card

What is the use of the Yellow Card?

The yellow card scheme is vital to help the MHRA monitor the safety of health care products in the UK and to ensure they are acceptably safe for patients that use them.

The scheme collects information on suspected problems or incident involving:

1. Side effect (adverse drugs reaction)
2. Medical device adverse incidents.
3. Defective medicines (drug that is not of acceptable quality).
4. Counterfeit or fake medication or medical devices.
5. Safety concern for cigarettes or their refill containers (liquid).

It recommends encouragement to adherence to medicines by supporting and involving people in the decision making. Report any form of adverse drug reactions to the health care providers' regulatory agency.

Z

Zimmer Walker

How do you use a Zimmer Walker?

1. Put your walker about one step ahead of you.
2. If your walker has wheels, roll it forward.
3. Make sure all four prongs or wheels are on the ground.
4. Look at where you are going.
5. Grip the top of the walker with both hands.
6. Keep your injured or weaker leg off the floor.
7. Move your stronger foot to the centre of the walker.
8. Move the walker forward to start the next step.

PRACTICE QUESTION FOR THE NMC CBT TEST.

1. **Symptoms of dehydrations are:**
A. Increased pulse rate and BP.
B. Increased pulse rate and decreased BP.
C. Decreased pulse rate and increased BP.
D. Decreased pulse rate and BP.

2. **A patient says, "I hate this cancer". According to Kubbler Ross stages of dying, the nurse understand that statement to refer as :**
A. Anger.
B. Denial.
C. Depression.
D. Bargaining.

3. **The Nurse is about to give digoxin tablet to a patient. And she noticed that the patient's heart rate was 58 beats/min. What is the best action to do?**
A. Give the medication because it is prescribed.
B. Give the medication as patient says this is his normal range of heart rate.
C. Hold the medication, document and report.
D. Hold the medication and beep the doctor.

4. **A patient is at the end stage of palliative care. Which among the following is not advisable?**
A. Giving analgesics and trying to relieve the symptoms.
B. Talk to family and friends to provide a psychological support.
C. Resuscitation.
D. Make the patient sit outside and engage in the activities he likes.

5. **A patient has tibia and fibula fracture. Which one of the following is not a symptom of Compartment syndrome?**
A. Pain not subsiding even after giving epidural analgesia.
B. Nausea and vomiting.
C. Tingling and numbness of the lower limb.
D. Cold extremities.

6. **The Nurse discloses a patient's information to a third party when:**
A. It is by the law/ order.
B. It is justified for public interest.
C. The media insists for disclosure.
D. It is by law/ order and justified for public interest.

7. **Holistic care is**
A. _____
B. _____
C. _____
D. _____

8. **Compassionate care is**
A. _____
B. _____
C. _____

9. **A Community Hospital in a local place should provide, what services?**
A. Rehabilitation, Physiotherapy, Psychiatry, Acute care.
B. Rehabilitation, Respite care, Acute and primary care, Physiotherapy, Psychiatry, Occupational therapy, Palliative care, Step down care for discharged patients.
C. Rehabilitation, Acute and Primary care, Occupational therapy, Step down care for discharged patients.
D. Rehabilitation, Respite care, Palliative care, Step down care for discharged patients.

10. **A patient with Lung cancer suffers from breathlessness, which should be the worst possible measure to take as a treatment?**
A. Crystal therapy by Traditional therapist.
B. Educating to control the breath by chest Physiotherapist.
C. Chest physiotherapy, by Physiotherapist.
D. Maintain the chest tube drainage system.

11. **A patient is on sub cute Fentanyl skin patch, common side effect of the Fentanyl overdose is:**
A. Fast and deep breathing, dizziness, sleepiness.
B. Slow and shallow breathing, dizziness, sleepiness.
C. Noisy and shallow breathing, dizziness, sleepiness.
D. Wheezes and shallow breathing, dizziness, sleepiness.

12. **What is the common cause of Airway Obstruction in an unconscious patient?**
A. Oropharyngeal tumour.
B. Laryngeal cyst.
C. Obstruction of foreign body.
D. Tongue falling back.

13. **Which of these is the most appropriate therapeutic communication?**
A. I'm sorry, your mother died.
B. I'm sorry; your mother has gone to Heaven.
C. I'm sorry; your mother is no longer with us.
D. I'm sorry, your mother passed on.

14. **The most common symptom of Type 1, Diabetes mellitus is**
A. Thirst.
B. Weight loss.
C. Ketoacidosis.
D. Diaphoresis.

15. What should a patient not do on using a Zimmer frame?
A. It can be used outside.
B. Don't carry any other thing with walker.
C. Push walker forward when using it.
D. Slide walker forward.

16. Immediately following Lumber Puncture to a client, she developed deterioration of consciousness, bradycardia, and increased Systolic blood pressure. What is the result of the manifestation of these symptoms?
A. Normal reaction.
B. Client has brain stem herniation.
C. Spinal headache.
D. Hyperflexia.

17. A drug 150g is prescribed and it is available as 5g per tablet. How many tablets are needed to be administered?
A. 30 tablets.
B. 15 tablets.
C. 3 tablets.
D. 5 tablets.

18. While changing the tubing on a patient with central line on the right Subclavian what should the nurse do to prevent complication?
A. Ask patient to breath normally.
B. Ask patient to hold the breath and bear down.
C. Inhale slowly.
D. Exhale slowly.

19. A new staff was careless about documenting patient's information and was reported by her colleague. What will be your action in solving this issue as the nurse manager?
A. Make her contact with the person that did induction programme.
B. Advice the colleague staff to help her.
C. In private call the staff and enquire about the problems in the new job area and clarify issues, as it is very important in the patients' care.
D. Report her carelessness to the Board.

20. A nurse assistant was found abusing an elderly patient verbally, what will be your action as a registered nurse?
A. Intervene immediately by stopping the staff, make sure that the patient is safe and report the incident to the authority.
B. Ignore the situation.
C. Report in the authority.
D. Enquire about the incident with the patient later.

21. What will be the first action to take against an incident of anaphylactic shock of a patient on IV Penicillin?
A. Stop the infusion immediately, call for help, make sure that the anaphylactic kit is available and don't leave the patient alone.
B. Reassure the patient and reduce the flow of the infusion.
C. Assess the patient and check vital signs.
D. Resuscitate by doing CPR.

22. Initial signs of phlebitis is
A. Hot and tender skin.
B. Signs of shock.
C. Cold skin with cyanosed nail bed.
D. Bleeding.

23. A patient asked an RN, "Can I tell you a secret?" What should be the RNs best response?
A. Yes because it develops trust which is central to the nursing practice.
B. Yes and will share it with the relevant medical team.
C. Yes I will share it with all the medical professionals who are supposed to know the secret.
D. Yes I will keep the secret because it is confidential.

24. A patient with COPD is discharged from the hospital, what advice should the nurse give to prevent exacerbation of the condition?
A. Advise the patient to take measures to quit smoking.
B. Advise the patient to do breathing exercise.
C. Teach purse lip breathing.
D. Advise to maintain adequate hydration.

25. A patient with dehydration has severe fluid volume deficit, which of the following signs will be indicated?
A. Hypotension.
B. A bounding pulse.
C. Increased urine output.
D. Increased respiratory rate.

26. A relative of a patient talks to the nurse over the phone and asks permission to come and visit the patient in the hospital. She admitted that she had few episodes of vomiting and diarrhea. What is the best response by the nurse?
A. Don't allow her to come and meet the patient.
B. Ask her to come and visit after 48hrs of recovery from the symptoms.
C. Advise her to sanitize the hands with hand sanitizer.
D. Advise her to treat herself.

27. A client has been diagnosed with atrial activity. Identify the ECG
A. Arterial fabrication.
B. Cardiac arrest.
C. Ventricular tachycardia.
D. Asystole.

28. A client is admitted at the psychiatric unit to be monitored for depression and suicidal behavior. On the 3rd day he seems to be very happy and is interacting with others, what could be this symptom concluded to be?
A. He has finalized his plan for suicide.
B. He's improving.
C. He has made new friends.
D. He is contemplating of committing suicide.

29. A drug 75ml is to be infused over half an hour. Calculate the milliters in an hour
A. 150m/hr.
B. 100m/hr.
C. 75m/hr.
D. 50m/hr.

30. A drug 8.25mg is ordered, it is available as 2.75mg. Calculate the dosage
A. 2 tablets
B. 3 tablets
C. 1 tablet
D. 4 tablets

31. Paracetamol 1gm is ordered but it is available as 500mg. How many tablets is needed to be administered?
A. 2 tablets.
B. 5 tablets.
C. 1 tablet.
D. 3 tablets.

32. What should be taught to a client about the use of Zimmer frame walker?
A. Move the affected leg first.
B. Move unaffected leg.
C. Move both legs together.
D. All of the above.

33. If an Oropharyngeal airway is inserted properly, what is the sign?
A. Airway obstruction.
B. Retching and vomiting.
C. Bradycardia.
D. Tachycardia.

34. A patient, who had stroke, sustained dysphagia. Which member of the interdisciplinary team should a nurse contact?
A. Physiotherapist.
B. Speech therapist.
C. Neurophysiologist.
D. Dietician.

35. A Community health nurse is taken history with the second year nursing student in a patient home. The nurse notice that a student nurse is not interested in the group discussion but was chatting on her phone. What is the ideal response from the Community health nurse?
A. Ask the student to leave the group.
B. Caution her at that moment by letting her know that such behaviour are not acceptable.
C. Inform to the principal.
D. Talk to her in private and let her be aware that such behavior is not expected of nurses.
E. Ask her to leave her phone and assist in what you are doing politely.

36. When a doctor, should prescribed a broad spectrum antibiotics?
A. On admission.
B. When septicaemia is suspected.
C. When the blood culture shows positive growth from organisms.
D. After obtaining blood samples for culture.

37. In the immediate post-operative period, what is the main priority?
A. Taking care of the airway.
B. Watching for blood lose.
C. Monitoring urine output.
D. Getting the consent.

38. How do you take an infected sheet for washing according to the UK standard?
A. Take infected linen in yellow bag for disposal.
B. Take in the red plastic bag that disintegrates in high temperature.
C. Use red linen bag that allows washing in high temperature.
D. Take the linen to the laundry.

39. You are the nurse at the Community Care Centre. An elderly patient complained to you that his neighbor is stealing money from him. He spends it on his shopping and sometimes the neighbor does not shop but rather keeps the money with him. What will you do?
A. Confront the neighbor when he visit you next time.
B. Remain quiet and ignore the complaint.
C. Request that the elderly talk to the Hospital Chaplin for further assistance.
D. Raise the complaint in the incident report form, investigate the matter and inform the concerned authorities.

40. A mentally health disordered client wants to leave the hospital. The medical team is not happy with his clinical condition according to the Mental Health Act. What will you do?
A. Let the client leave the hospital as long as he does not possess any threat to the public or visibly ill.
B. Inform the security to hold the patient and do not let him go away.
C. Inform the police.
D. Counsel the patient to stay back in the hospital for him to get much.

41. What is the purpose of Clinical Audit?
A. It helps to understand the functioning and effectiveness of nursing activities.
B. Helps to understand the outcomes and process of medical and surgical procedures.
C. Helps to identify areas of improvement in the system pertaining to nursing and medical practitioners.
D. Helps to understand medical outcomes and process only.

42. While brushing the teeth of a client the nurse observed that the client has bleeding gums. The nurse understands that the cause of this gingivitis is
A. Poor flossing.
B. Poor tarter removal.
C. Infection.
D. Poor nutrition.
E. All of the above.

43. Who among the patients with these symptoms listed below are more prone to Coronary artery disease?
A. Hypotension, smoker, DM, obese women, non-sedentary lifestyle.
B. Hypotension, smoker, DM, obese men with, non-sedentary lifestyle.
C. Hypertension, smoker, obese men, sedentary lifestyle.
D. Hypertension, obese women, diabetes, sedentary lifestyle.

44. What type of drugs causes most of the falls in older patients?
A. Hypnotics.
B. Loop diuretics.
C. Beta blockers.
D. Non-steroidal anti-inflammatory drugs.

45. Which condition is not a cause of diarrhea?
A. Ulcerative colitis.
B. Intestinal obstruction.
C. Hashimotos disease.
D. Food allergy.

46. Which among the following is a cause of Hemorrhoids?
A. High fiber rich diet.
B. Non-processed food.
C. Straining while passing stools.
D. Unsaturated fats in the diet.

47. While teaching a patient to walk in a Zimmer walker, which is the most appropriate advice?
A. Lift the walker 10 inches forward then take 2 steps and come in the middle.
B. Slide the walker 10 inches forward then take small steps to maintain balance.
C. Lift the walker 5 minutes forward then take 1 step and come in the middle.
D. Slide walker 5 minutes backward and change with the leg.

48. A patient with Clostridium deficile has bloody mucoid stool due to which of the following conditions?
A. Ulcerative colitis.
B. Chrohn's disease.
C. Inflammatory bowel disease.
D. Colitis.

49. A patient is given penicillin tablet. After 12 hours the patient developed itches, rashes and shortness of breath. What could be the reason?
A. Speed shock.
B. Allergic reaction.
C. Anaphylactic reaction.
D. Bradycardia.

50. For every patient admitted in the ward, discharge planning should be done at which time of the process?
A. Within 24 hours of admission.
B. When patient tells he wants to leave.
C. When the family request for a discharge.
D. Immediately after the doctor's order for discharge.

51. When does the proliferation phase start in wound healing?
A. 10-24 days.
B. Within minutes.
C. 1-2 days.
D. 25 days or more.

52. A patient on Post-op was found crying, she said that the pain has not reduced even after given an analgesic. What is your next action as a nurse?
A. Call the doctor.
B. Give a semi-reclined position to the patient.
C. Give a heat pad for application.
D. Provide a glass of water.

53. A patient is getting a discharge with continuing Oxygen therapy, 2 Litres through the Nasal cannula. When you visited the patient you found out that the patient is dyspneic, anxious and frightened. What is the best action for the nurse to take?
A. Administer tab. or morph which is prescribed as PNO.
B. Try to calm down the patient.
C. Decrease the level of Oxygen.
D. Increase the level of Oxygen.

54. You have just finished dressing a wound of a patient with leg ulcer and you observed that the patient was depressed and withdrawn. You asked the patient if everything was okay. She said "yes". What should be your next action?
A. Say "I observe you don't seem as usual. Are you sure you are okay?"
B. Say "Cheer up, shall I make a cup of tea for you?"
C. Accept her response and leave to attend to other patients.
D. Inform the doctor about the change of behavior.

55. The proper eye administration installation is
A. Supine.
B. Sit up and head tilt backwards.
C. Sit up and lean forward.
D. Standing.

56. While gaining consent the nurse should assess for
A. Capacity.
B. Understanding.
C. Emotions.
D. Sensitivity.

57. Which position is suitable for the patient after abdominal Paracentesis?
A. Supine with knees bent.
B. Supine with head raised 40-50 degrees.
C. Sitting at the edge of the bed.
D. Prone.

58. What is the most serious complication after liver biopsy within 24hrs?
A. Nausea and vomiting.
B. Pain at the site of biopsy.
C. Back pain.
D. Bleeding.

59. Which of the following is an indication for Intra pleural chest drain insertion?
A. Pneumothorax.
B. Tuberculosis.
C. Asthma.
D. Malignancy of the lungs.

60. Which is the most suitable site for assessing oedema?
A. Foot/Ankle.
B. Clavicle.
C. Sternum.
D. Scapular.

61. Which is the most common sign of dehydration in older adults?
A. Reduced skin turgor.
B. Bruises.
C. Skin lesions.
D. Pale/Cyanosis.

62. A Jewish patient in a critical condition refuses the blood transfusion and states that his religion is against it. What should the nurse do?
A. Ignore client's wishes and give him blood.
B. Tell the patient's relatives to take decision.
C. Accept the client's wishes.
D. Force the client to give consent.

63. The important advice that should be given to a patient on medication (allopurinol) should be to?
A. Drink plenty of fluids.
B. Take analgesics.
C. Take whenever patient demand for it.
D. Give with herbal preparation.

64. Protective diets are full of anti-oxidants and are helpful in diseased conditions, which of the following can be included in a protective diet?
A. Tomatoes, carrots and broccoli.
B. Beef fish and chicken.
C. Eggs dairy and cheese.
D. Rice beans and pasta.

65. You are caring for a Hindu client and it's time for drug administration, the client refuses to take the capsule saying that animal products might have been used in producing the drugs, what is the appropriate action for the nurse to perform?
A. She will not administer but document the omissions in the patients chart.
B. The nurse will ignore the clients request and administer forcefully.
C. The nurse will open the capsule and administer the powdered drug.
D. The nurse will have to collaborate with the pharmacist to determine if the capsule is suitable for vegetarians.

66. There is a Chinese client in your care and the relatives of the client insisted on bringing their own food for the client, what is the appropriate thing for the nurse to do?
A. Accept their wishes under Western Foods and Cultural differences considerations.
B. Refuse the client's wish as the food might carry infection.
C. Ask the next of kin to bring in the food and hand it to the dietary unit for approval.
D. Tell them it is not accepted, firmly.

67. A patient wants to leave hospital against medical advice. The doctors are concerned about the patient's competent under the mental capacity act. What should the nurse do?
A. Let the patient go, he is competent and in his full sense.
B. Call for police.
C. Restrain the patient.
D. Call the security and make the patient stay until the doctor complete their assessment.

68. A terminally ill patient tells the nurse that he doesn't want CPR. What should the nurse do?
A. Force the patient to have the CPR that it is very important.
B. Ask the relatives to talk to the patient.
C. Tell the patient that his decision is absolutely right.
D. Explain to him about advanced directives.

69. A patient is in hypovolemic shock. All are the symptoms except
A. Bleeding.
B. Diaphoresis.
C. Cold clammy skin.
D. Confusion.

70. What is Advocacy according to NHS Trust?

A. It is a set of rules or a promise that limits access or places restrictions on certain types of information.

B. This is the divulging or provision of access to data.

C. It is the response to the suffering of others that motivates a desire to help.

D. It is taking action to help people say what they want, secure their rights, represent their interests and obtain the services they need.

NMC CBT, PRACTICE TEST ANSWERS.

1. B – Increased pulse rate and decreased BP.

2. A – Anger.

3. C – Hold the medication, document and report.

4. C – Resuscitation.

5. B – Nausea.

6. A – It is by the law/ order.

7. A – Physical; B – Social; C – Psychological; D – Spiritual.

8. A – Care; B – Dignity; C – Respect.

9. A – Rehabilitation, Physiotherapy, Psychiatry, Acute care.

10. B – Educating to control the breath by chest physiotherapy.

11. B – Slow and shallow breathing, dizziness, sleepiness.

12. D – Tongue falling back.

13. D – I'm sorry, your mother passed on.

14. A – Thirst.

15. C – Push walker forward when using it.

16. B – Client has brain stem herniation.

17. A – 30 tablets.

18. B – Ask patient to hold the breath and bear down.

19. C –In private call the staff and enquire about the problems in the new job area and clarify issues, as it is very important in the patients' care.

20. A – Intervene immediately by stopping the staff, make sure the patient is safe and reportthe incident to the authority.

21. A - Stop the infusion immediately, call for help, make sure that the anaphylactic kit is available and don't leave the patient alone.

22. A – Hot and tender skin.

23. D – Yes, I will keep the secret because it is confidential.

24. A – Advise the patient to take measures to quit smoking.

25. A – Hypotension.

26. B – Ask her to come and visit after 48 hours of recovery from the symptoms.

27. A – Arterial fibrillation.

28. A – He has finalized his plain for suicide.

29. A – 150m/hr.

30. B – 3 tablets.

31. A – 2 tablets.

32. A – Move the affected leg first.

33. B – Retching and vomiting.

34. B – Speech therapist.

35. E – Ask her to leave her phone and assist in what you are doing.

36. D – After obtaining blood samples for culture.
37. A – Taking care of the airway.

38. B – Take in the red plastic bag that disintegrates in high temperature.

39. D – Raise the complaint in the incident report form, investigate the matter and inform the concerned authorities.

40. A – Let the client leave the hospital as long as he does not possess any threat to the public or is visibly ill.

41. C – Helps to identify areas of improvement in the system pertaining nursing and medical practitioners.

42. E – All of the above.

43. C, D – Hypertension, smoker, obese men, sedentary lifestyle; D- Hypertension, obese women, diabetes, sedentary lifestyle.

44. A – Hypnotics.

45. B – Intestinal obstruction.

46. C – Straining while passing stool.

47. B – Slide the walker 10 inches forward, then take small steps to maintain balance.

48. D – Colitis.

49. C – Anaphylactic reaction.

50. A – within 24 hours of admission.

51. A – 10-24 days.

52. A – Call the doctor.

53. D – Increase the level of Oxygen.

54. A – Say "I observe you don't seem as usual. Are you sure you are okay?"

55. B – Sit up and head tilt backwards.

56. B – Understanding.

57. B– Supine with head raised 40- 50 cm.

58. D – Bleeding.

59. A – Pneumothorax.

60. A – Foot/Ankle

61. A – Reduced skin turgor.

62. C – Accept the client's wishes.

63. A – Drink plenty water.

64. A – Tomatoes, carrots and broccoli.

65. D – The nurse will have to collaborate with the pharmacist to determine if the capsule is suitable for vegetarians.

66. A – Accept their wishes under Western Foods and Cultural differences considerations.

67. A – Let the patient go, he is competent and in his full sense.

68. D – Explain to him about advance directives.

69. B, C, D: B - Diaphoresis; C - Cold clammy skin, D – Confusion.

70. D – It is taking action to help people say what they want, secure their rights, represent their interests and obtain the services they need.

REFERENCES.

Linda Anne Silvestri. (2017).Saunders Comprehensive Review for the NCLEX-RN Examination (ed 7). St Louis, Missouri: Elsevier; 208-211.

Davis, charlotte BSN, RN, CCRN; Nursing Made Incredibly Easy: March/April 2015 – Volume 13 – Issue 2 – P4.

Davidson, N; Williams, K (2009). Compassion in nursing 1: identifying and measuring these quality. Nursing Times; 105: 36, earl online publication.

Dougherty, L., & Lister S. (2015). The Royal Marsden Manual of Clinical Nursing Proceedure. The Royal Marsden NHS Foundation Trust. (ed 9; Professional edition). Willey Blackwell.

Online References

National Council of States Board of Nursing. (2014).Professional Boundaries.   (Website); www.ncsbn.org/professionalboundaries_complete.pdf

NHS Choices. (2017). Diarrhoea. (Website); www.nhs.uk

National Institute for Health and Care Excellence. (2017). Managing Medicines for adults Receiving Social Care in the Community. (Website); www.nice.org.uk/guidance

Healthy and Safety Executive. (2016). Patient Safety. (Website); www.hse.gov.uk

Nursing and Midwifery Council. (2016).The code for Nurses and Midwives. (Website); www.nmc.org.uk/standards

Nursing and Midwifery Council. (2017). Confidentiality; Disclosure; Raising concern. (Website); www.nmc.org.uk/raisingconcerns

Centre for Disease Control and Prevention (2019). U.S Department of Health and Human Services. https://www.cdc.gov/coronavirus/2019-ncov/symptoms-testing/symptoms.html

World Health Organisation (WHO) (2019). Coronavirus Disease (COVID-19) Pandemic. https://ww.who.int/emergencies/diseases/novel-coronavirus-2019.

Made in the USA
Columbia, SC
06 October 2024

43764859R00090